Consultations in Liver Disease

Editor

STEVEN L. FLAMM

CLINICS IN LIVER DISEASE

www.liver.theclinics.com

Consulting Editor
NORMAN GITLIN

November 2017 • Volume 21 • Number 4

ELSEVIER

1600 John F. Kennedy Boulevard • Suite 1800 • Philadelphia, Pennsylvania, 19103-2899

http://www.theclinics.com

CLINICS IN LIVER DISEASE Volume 21, Number 4
November 2017 ISSN 1089-3261, ISBN-13: 978-0-323-54885-4

Editor: Kerry Holland
Developmental Editor: Meredith Madeira

Clinics in Liver Disease (ISSN 1089-3261) is published quarterly by Elsevier Inc., 360 Park Avenue South, New York, NY 10010-1710. Months of issue are February, May, August, and November. Business and Editorial Offices: 1600 John F. Kennedy Blvd., Ste. 1800, Philadelphia, PA 19103-2899. Customer Service Office: 3251 Riverport Lane, Maryland Heights, MO 63043. Periodicals postage paid at New York, NY and additional mailing offices. Subscription prices are $281.00 per year (U.S. individuals), $100.00 per year (U.S. student/resident), $476.00 per year (U.S. institutions), $403.00 per year (international individuals), $200.00 per year (international student/resident), $590.00 per year (international instituitions), $347.00 per year (Canadian individuals), $200.00 per year (Canadian student/resident), and $590.00 per year (Canadian institutions). Foreign air speed delivery is included in all *Clinics* subscription prices. All prices are subject to change without notice. **POSTMASTER:** Send address changes to *Clinics in Liver Disease*, Elsevier Health Sciences Division, Subscription Customer Service, 3251 Riverport Lane, Maryland Heights, MO 63043. **Customer Service: Telephone: 1-800-654-2452 (U.S. and Canada); 314-447-8871 (outside U.S. and Canada). Fax: 314-447-8029. E-mail: journalscustomer service-usa@elsevier.com (for print support); journalsonlinesupport-usa@elsevier.com (for online support).**

Reprints. For copies of 100 or more of articles in this publication, please contact the Commercial Reprints Department, Elsevier Inc., 360 Park Avenue South, New York, NY 10010-1710. Tel.: 212-633-3874; Fax: 212-633-3820; E-mail: reprints@elsevier.com.

Clinics in Liver Disease is covered in *MEDLINE/PubMed (Index Medicus)*, Science Citation Index Expanded, Journal Citation Reports/Science Edition, and Current Contents/Clinical Medicine.

Contributors

CONSULTING EDITOR

NORMAN GITLIN, MD, FRCP (LONDON), FRCPE (EDINBURGH), FAASLD, FACP, FACG
Formerly, Professor, Department of Medicine, Chief of Hepatology, Emory University, Currently, Consultant, Atlanta Gastroenterology Associates, Atlanta, Georgia, USA

EDITOR

STEVEN L. FLAMM, MD
Professor, Department of Medicine, Division of Gastroenterology and Hepatology, Northwestern University Feinberg School of Medicine, Chicago, Illinois, USA

AUTHORS

JOSEPH AHN, MD
Associate Professor, Department of Medicine, Division of Gastroenterology and Hepatology, Oregon Health & Science University, Portland, Oregon, USA

ROBERT S. BROWN Jr, MD, MPH
Gladys and Roland Harriman Professor of Medicine, Vice Chair, Transitions of Care, Clinical Chief, Division of Gastroenterology and Hepatology, Center for Liver Disease and Transplantation, Weill Cornell Medicine, New York, New York, USA

CHALERMRAT BUNCHORNTAVAKUL, MD
Assistant Professor, Division of Gastroenterology and Hepatology, Department of Medicine, Rajavithi Hospital, College of Medicine, Rangsit University, Bangkok, Thailand; Division of Gastroenterology and Hepatology, Department of Medicine, Hospital of the University of Pennsylvania, University of Pennsylvania, Philadelphia, Pennsylvania, USA

BLAIRE E. BURMAN, MD
Assistant Professor, Division of Gastroenterology and Hepatology, Virginia Mason Medical Center, Seattle, Washington, USA

HALEY BUSH, MSPH
Betty & Guy Beatty Center for Integrated Research, Inova Health System, Inova Fairfax Hospital, Falls Church, Virginia, USA

AMANDA CHEUNG, MD
Fellow, Division of Gastroenterology and Hepatology, Northwestern University Feinberg School of Medicine, Chicago, Illinois, USA

RENU DHANASEKARAN, MD
Instructor, Department of Medicine, Stanford University School of Medicine, Palo Alto, California, USA

STEVEN L. FLAMM, MD
Professor, Department of Medicine, Division of Gastroenterology and Hepatology, Northwestern University Feinberg School of Medicine, Chicago, Illinois, USA

PEGAH GOLABI, MD
Betty & Guy Beatty Center for Integrated Research, Inova Health System, Inova Fairfax Hospital, Falls Church, Virginia, USA

GREGORY J. GORES, MD
Professor, Department of Medicine, Division of Gastroenterology and Hepatology, Mayo Clinic, Rochester, Minnesota, USA

ANDREA A. GOSSARD, APRN, CNP
Associate Professor, Department of Medicine, Division of Gastroenterology and Hepatology, Mayo Clinic, Rochester, Minnesota, USA

IRA M. JACOBSON, MD
Professor of Medicine, Chairman, Department of Medicine, Division of Digestive Diseases, Mount Sinai Beth Israel, Icahn School of Medicine at Mount Sinai, New York, New York, USA

MANAN A. JHAVERI, MD, MPH
Transplant Hepatology Fellow, Department of Organ Transplant & Liver Center, Liver Care Network and Organ Care Research, Swedish Medical Center, Seattle, Washington, USA

KRIS V. KOWDLEY, MD, FACP, FAASLD
Director, Department of Organ Transplant & Liver Center, Liver Care Network and Organ Care Research, Swedish Medical Center, Seattle, Washington, USA

PAUL Y. KWO, MD
Professor, Department of Medicine, Director of Hepatology, Stanford University School of Medicine, Palo Alto, California, USA

JOSH LEVITSKY, MD, MS
Professor, Division of Gastroenterology and Hepatology, Northwestern University Feinberg School of Medicine, Chicago, Illinois, USA

HARIPRIYA MADDUR, MD
Assistant Professor, Department of Medicine, Division of Gastroenterology and Hepatology, Northwestern University Feinberg School of Medicine, Chicago, Illinois, USA

ARNAB MITRA, MD
Fellow, Department of Medicine, Division of Gastroenterology and Hepatology, Oregon Health & Science University, Portland, Oregon, USA

K. RAJENDER REDDY, MD
Ruimy Family President's Distinguished Professor of Medicine and Surgery, Division of Gastroenterology and Hepatology, Department of Medicine, Hospital of the University of Pennsylvania, University of Pennsylvania, Philadelphia, Pennsylvania, USA

MICHAEL L. SCHILSKY, MD, FAASLD
Professor, Department of Medicine and Surgery, Sections of Digestive Diseases and Transplantation and Immunology, Yale School of Medicine, New Haven, Connecticut, USA

EMILY A. SCHONFELD, MD
Transplant Hepatology Fellow, Center for Liver Disease and Transplantation, Columbia University Medical Center, New York, New York, USA

ILAN S. WEISBERG, MD
Assistant Professor, Department of Medicine, Division of Digestive Diseases, Mount Sinai Beth Israel, Icahn School of Medicine at Mount Sinai, New York, New York, USA

ZOBAIR M. YOUNOSSI, MD, MPH, FACG, FACP, AGAF
Department of Medicine, Center for Liver Disease, Betty & Guy Beatty Center for Integrated Research, Inova Health System, Inova Fairfax Hospital, Falls Church, Virginia, USA

Contents

postulated to be multifactorial. Diagnosis in adults is primarily by exclusion, eliminating other causes of chronic liver disease or cirrhosis, and other factors seen in critically ill or postoperative patients on TPN. Principal treatment is avoiding TPN. If this is not feasible, research supports fish oil–based lipid emulsions in TPN formulations to reduce risk and progression of PNALD. With liver and intestinal failure, liver and intestine transplantation is an option.

Gastroenterologists and hepatologists will encounter oncology patients who develop abnormal liver tests, patients with hepatic malignancies, and patients with acute and chronic liver disease who require chemotherapy or immediate evaluation. Chemotherapy can cause liver injury owing to toxic effects or idiosyncratic reactions. Immune checkpoint inhibitors may be associated with autoimmune-mediated liver toxicities. Veno-occlusive disease requires immediate evaluation. Nodular regenerative hyperplasia is a chronic progressive disorder. Screening and prophylaxis for reactivation of hepatitis B is important to minimize complications in patients receiving chemotherapy. Patients with metastatic lesions can undergo resection or ablation. Hepatic injury may occur in those receiving radiation-based therapies.

Primary biliary cholangitis (PBC) is an autoimmune liver disease characterized by chronic granulomatous lymphocytic cholangitis of the small bile ducts. PBC was a leading indication for liver transplantation in the United States; with early diagnosis and treatment, most patients with PBC have a normal life expectancy. Pathogenesis involves inflammatory damage of bile duct epithelium secondary to innate and adaptive immune responses, and toxicity from accumulated bile acids. Cholestasis and disease progression can lead to cirrhosis. Extrahepatic complications include dyslipidemia, metabolic bone disease, and fat-soluble vitamin deficiency. Ursodeoxycholic acid is a well-established therapy. Novel targeted therapeutics are being developed.

Primary sclerosing cholangitis (PSC) is a chronic, idiopathic biliary tract disease characterized by segmental strictures. The disease is progressive with no proven treatments and may eventually lead to cirrhosis and endstage liver disease. Abrupt changes in liver biochemistries, pain, and/or cholangitis may suggest a dominant stricture amenable to endoscopic therapy or the development of cholangiocarcinoma. Patients with PSC are at increased risk of cholangiocarcinoma. There is a strong association

with withdrawal strategies, and more optimal management of long-term risks, such as malignancy, cardiovascular disease, and renal failure. In addition, now that short-term results (<1 year) have improved significantly, there will be a shift toward improving long-term patient and graft survival, as well as a focus on primary care preventive strategies.

CLINICS IN LIVER DISEASE

THE CLINICS ARE AVAILABLE ONLINE!
Access your subscription at:
www.theclinics.com

Preface

Consultations in Liver Disease

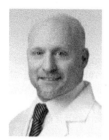

Steven L. Flamm, MD
Editor

Gastroenterology practitioners often are requested to opine on patients with complicated liver-related issues in both the outpatient and the inpatient setting. The problems are frequently uncommon and occasionally life threatening. Rapid advances in the field may be difficult to follow for providers in a busy Gastroenterology practice. This issue of *Clinics in Liver Disease*, entitled Consultations in Liver Disease, is the third in a series. The first, entitled Approach to Consultation for Patients with Liver Disease published in May 2012, and the second, entitled Consultations in Liver Disease published in February 2015, include a series of liver-related topics that Gastroenterology clinicians encounter in practice. Each discussion provides a succinct, clinically oriented approach of how to address common liver-related problems. This issue of *Clinics in Liver Disease* introduces a number of additional topics to aid the clinician in caring for inpatients and outpatients with liver disease.

Advances in the care of patients with chronic hepatitis C virus (HCV) infection have been nothing short of stunning in recent years. The vast majority of patients are now cured with therapies that are easy to administer for the Gastroenterology provider. However, some issues remain. Dr Maddur and I review the data on patients with HCV genotype 3 and how it differs from the others and approaches on how to treat it. Irrespective of the genotype, a small number of patients fail therapy with direct-acting antiviral agents (DAAs). Most have resistance to one or more classes of DAAs. Drs Weisberg and Jacobson then discuss the "ins and outs" of HCV resistance, its impact on therapeutic response, and how to test for it.

One of the recent advances in the field of Hepatology has been the identification of specific genetic abnormalities for different disease states. Many genetic tests are available. Drs Schonfeld and Brown outline a spectrum of genetic tests for liver disease problems, including how and when to order them.

A common difficult inpatient consultation for the Gastroenterologist includes the impact of total parenteral nutrition on the liver. Drs Mitra and Ahn discuss how to

Clin Liver Dis 21 (2017) xiii–xiv
http://dx.doi.org/10.1016/j.cld.2017.08.016
1089-3261/17/© 2017 Published by Elsevier Inc.

evaluate and manage such patients. Oncology patients frequently have liver issues, either from the disease process or from medications, including chemotherapy. Drs Dhanasekaran and Kwo discuss a clinical approach for assessing these patients.

Primary biliary cholangitis (PBC) and primary sclerosing cholangitis (PSC), autoimmune diseases that affect the liver, are uncommon but not rare. Gastroenterology practitioners will likely be consulted to evaluate patients with these problems. There have been new advances in therapy and management. Drs Burman, Jhaveri, and Kowdley elaborate on recent advances in the therapy of PBC, and Drs Gossard and Gores outline evaluation and management strategies for PSC.

The most common liver disease in the United States is fatty liver/nonalcoholic steatohepatitis (NAFLD). There have been recent developments in the understanding of NAFLD, and extensive efforts are underway in the research setting to provide new therapies for this unmet medical need. Drs Golabi, Bush, and Younossi report on an approach to evaluate these patients and discuss areas of investigation that it is hoped will lead to new options for therapy in the near future.

Dr Schilsky details how to evaluate and manage patients with Wilson disease, and Drs Bunchorntavakul and Reddy discuss the current state-of-the-art for identifying and caring for patients with acute liver failure.

Finally, life-saving liver transplantation is indicated in patients with complications of end-stage liver disease. These patients are on long-term immunosuppression and may be referred back to the referring Gastroenterologist after recovery from surgery. Drs Cheung and Levitsky provide an excellent clinically focused review on issues that occur in the post–liver transplantation setting oriented to the Gastroenterology practitioner.

This issue of *Clinics in Liver Disease* complements the previous two issues by providing additional topics that will help the clinical practitioner develop a framework to address difficult and rapidly changing aspects of liver disease in the outpatient and inpatient setting that were not discussed previously.

I would like to thank Dr Norman Gitlin for offering me the opportunity to serve as the editor for this issue of *Clinics in Liver Disease*. Furthermore, I would like to thank Kerry Holland and Meredith Madeira for their tireless assistance in preparing the articles for publication.

Steven L. Flamm, MD
Division of Gastroenterology and Hepatology
Northwestern University
Feinberg School of Medicine
676 North St Clair, 19th Floor
Chicago, IL 60611, USA

E-mail address:
s-flamm@northwestern.edu

Hepatitis C Genotype 3 Infection
Pathogenesis and Treatment Horizons

Haripriya Maddur, MD*, Steven L. Flamm, MD

KEYWORDS

- Hepatitis C • Genotype 3 • Hepatocellular carcinoma • Hepatic steatosis
- Accelerated fibrosis

KEY POINTS

- Hepatitis C genotype 3 infection is associated with increased late-stage liver events, accelerated hepatic fibrosis, and hepatocellular carcinoma.
- Infection with genotype 3 infection has been linked to hepatic steatosis thought to be related to direct viral protein effect on hepatocytes.
- With the advent of direct-acting antiviral therapies, infection with genotype 3 has been found to be more difficult to treat as compared with other genotypes.

INTRODUCTION

Chronic hepatitis C virus (HCV) infection is a global epidemic affecting approximately 170 million people. It is a major cause of cirrhosis, observed in approximately one-quarter of those chronically infected.[1] The mortality related to decompensated cirrhosis is high, with a 5-year survival of approximately 50%.[2] Furthermore, HCV is the leading indication for liver transplantation in the Western world.[3] Six major genotypes (GTs) have been identified worldwide, with GTs 1, 2, and 3 accounting for most identified infections within the United States.[4]

It has been clear for many years that the different GTs respond differently to interferon-alfa-based medical regimens. Sustained virologic response (SVR) rates with pegylated interferon and ribavirin for GT 1 infection were less than 50%, and 48 weeks of therapy were required.[5] Infection with GTs 2 and 3, accounting for approximately one-third of patients in the United States, was easier to treat with SVR rates exceeding 70% with only 24 weeks of therapy recommended.[6] With the advent of noninterferon-based therapies (direct-acting antiviral agents

The authors have nothing to disclose.
Division of Gastroenterology and Hepatology, Northwestern University Feinberg School of Medicine, 676 North St Clair, 19th Floor, Chicago, IL 60611, USA
* Corresponding author.
E-mail address: HMADDUR@nm.org

[DAA]), however, GT 3 infection has become more difficult to treat. GT 3 subjects with some regimens require an extended duration of therapy, and lower SVR rates are observed, particularly in patients with cirrhosis and who have been previously treated with interferon-alfa-based regimens.

Unlike the long-standing well-known different treatment responses for the various GTs, until recently, it has been thought that the natural history of the different GTs was similar. However, evidence has been emerging that there are differences. Infection with GT 3 infection, in particular, has been associated with an increase in mortality when compared with GT 1. Specifically, there is an increased risk of hepatocellular carcinoma and a higher risk of late-stage liver events.[6–8] Central to the aggressive natural history and relative resistance to treatment of GT 3 HCV infection is its association with hepatic steatosis leading to increased necroinflammatory activity via oxidative stress.[6]

A factor implicated in lower treatment response rates is the presence of baseline and treatment-emergent resistance-associated variants (RAVs), also called resistance-associated substitutions. NS5A RAVs are particularly problematic. When detected, these markers denote those who are at increased risk of virologic relapse and may identify those patients who require a longer duration of therapy or benefit from the addition of ribavirin. Lower response rates are observed in patients with cirrhosis and in patients who are treatment experienced. Patients who are cirrhotic and treatment experienced have the lowest treatment response rates.[9]

This article reviews current data on the natural history and treatment approaches to HCV GT 3.

DEMOGRAPHICS

GT 3 infection is the second most common hepatitis C GT, accounting for approximately 30% of infections. Worldwide, an estimated 54.3 million individuals are infected with HCV GT 3.[10] The prevalence of GT 3 infection is highest in Southeast Asia, accounting for approximately 40% of infections, primarily in India and Pakistan.[11] Within the United States, the prevalence of GT 3 infection is slightly lower, accounting for approximately 12% of infections. GT 3 infection is unique in that it has been associated with accelerated hepatic fibrosis and hepatic steatosis.[12]

Changes in host metabolism and insulin resistance have been identified in HCV-infected individuals, thus leading to hepatic steatosis.[13] GT 3 infection has been associated with a higher incidence of hepatic steatosis when compared with all other GTs (73% vs 50%).[14–17] The mechanism is thought to involve a direct viral protein effect on hepatocytes. In vitro studies have found that protein expression in GT 3 leads to a three-fold increase in intracellular triglyceride accumulation when compared with other GTs.[18] The development of hepatic steatosis results in accelerated development of hepatic fibrosis.[19] In one study, patients with HCV infection with significant steatosis were noted to have elevated fibrosis scores when compared with those with less steatosis. When compared with individuals infected with GT 1 and 4, subjects infected with GT 3 have been found to have a faster rate of hepatic fibrosis progression over time.[20]

Studies of GT 3–infected subjects have noted a correlation of elevated viral load with increased hepatic fibrosis.[21] Moreover, in patients with GT 3 infection, eradication of virus has been found to improve and, in some cases, resolve steatosis. This has not been observed in GT 1 infection.[6,14,19,22] Within the posttransplant setting, patients with GT 3 have been found to have histologic recurrence of hepatic steatosis following orthotopic liver transplantation.[23]

When patients with GT 3 infection were compared with those with GT 1, 2, or 4 infection, those with GT 3 were found to have an increased progression to cirrhosis at a younger age when compared with GT 1–infected individuals. In this study, GT 3–infected subjects were also found to have a higher incidence of hepatocellular carcinoma.[24] These findings corroborated previous retrospective data showing an increased risk of hepatocellular carcinoma in GT 3–infected individuals when compared with all other GTs (34% vs 17%).[7] GT 3 infection is also associated with increased rates of decompensated cirrhosis, liver-related hospitalization, and death when compared with GT 1– and GT 2–infected individuals.[8]

TREATMENT
Interferon-Alfa-Based Regimens

Historically, treatment recommendations for GT 2 and GT 3 infection were coupled together. In the era of interferon-alfa-based regimens, for many years, a 24-week course of pegylated interferon and low-dose ribavirin (800 mg) was recommended for GT 2 and GT 3, whereas 48 weeks of therapy was recommended for GT 1 with pegylated interferon and weight-based ribavirin (1000–1200 mg per day in divided doses).[25,26] When peginterferon alfa-2a plus ribavirin was compared with peginterferon alfa-2a alone versus interferon alfa-2b alone, treatment response rates were noted to be improved with peginterferon alfa-2a plus ribavirin (56%), versus 44% and 36%, respectively. When treatment response rates for GT 1 infection were compared with response rates for GT 2 or 3 infection collectively, response rates were better for GT 2 and 3 (76% vs 46%).[27]

In a subsequent trial, peginterferon alfa-2a and weight-based ribavirin therapy yielded a higher overall SVR rate of 63%. When individuals with GT 1 infection were compared with those with GT 2 and 3 infection, SVR rates with 48 weeks of therapy were 52% versus 80%. In this study, for GT 2– and 3–infected individuals, SVR rates were 84% versus 80% with 24 versus 48 weeks therapy, respectively. Additionally, although patients with GT 1 infection had higher response rates with standard weight-based ribavirin compared with a low, flat dose, response rates with weight-based ribavirin dosing did not benefit GT 2 and 3 infection compared with the low, flat dose.[28] Similar response rates were reported in another trial with peginterferon alfa2b and ribavirin with SVR rates of 42% for GT 1–infected patients versus 80% for patients with GT 2 and 3 infection after 48 weeks of therapy.[29] Only weight-based ribavirin dosing was investigated with this peginterferon alfa product. Nevertheless, the general recommendation for GT 2 or 3 infection was treatment with a 24-week course of peginterferon alfa plus a flat dose of 800 mg ribavirin. Although initially it was thought that GT 2 and 3 had similar response rates to one another, it soon became clear that GT 3–infected patients had lower SVR rates, largely secondary to an increased rate of virologic relapse.[30,31]

It should also be noted that treatment with interferon-alfa-based therapies is limited by an unfavorable side effect profile, including influenza-like symptoms, psychiatric effects, such as depression, and cytopenias, among others, prohibiting widespread use of these regimens. Additionally, ribavirin use is associated with hemolytic anemia, lymphopenia, hyperuricemia, and rash. Ribavirin is also teratogenic, necessitating the use of contraception while on therapy and for 6 months thereafter. Furthermore, ribavirin is cleared by the kidney, mandating caution with use in patients with renal impairment.[25] Yet, pegylated interferon alfa once weekly and ribavirin 800 mg daily for 24 weeks constituted the standard of care for HCV GT 3 in the United States until late 2013. In some parts of the world, this regimen remains the standard because of lack of availability of newer regimens and cost considerations.

Direct-Acting Antiviral Agents

In recent years, oral direct DAAs were approved for treatment of HCV. The first agents were the protease inhibitors, boceprevir and telaprevir, approved in the United States in 2011 in combination with pegylated interferon alfa and ribavirin for treatment of GT 1. These agents added significant toxicity to the standard interferon-alfa-based regimen, although higher SVR rates were observed in GT 1. Unfortunately, the new regimens were still suboptimal for GT 1, and they were not approved for therapies of other GTs, including GT 3. New oral regimens with DAAs were sought.

Studies with DAAs in GT 3 were first reported using sofosbuvir, an oral nucleotide analogue inhibitor of the HCV NS5B polymerase. Sofosbuvir, when used in combination with ribavirin within the context of an interferon-free regimen, was found to be effective in GT 2 and 3 patients, although there were lower SVR rates in GT 3–infected individuals. The FISSION trial randomized patients with GT 2 or 3 infection to therapy with sofosbuvir, 400 mg daily, plus ribavirin, 800 mg, in divided doses daily for 12 weeks or peginterferon alpha-2a plus ribavirin (the previous standard) for 24 weeks. In this study, overall SVR rates at 12 weeks following treatment completion were statistically equivalent between the two regimens, specifically 67% in each group. However, when GT 3 patients were evaluated separately, response rates were lower, 56% in patients receiving sofosbuvir plus ribavirin versus 63% in patients receiving peginterferon plus ribavirin. Fatigue, headache, nausea, and insomnia were seen in both treatment groups. However, the incidence of side effects was markedly less in the sofosbuvir regimen treatment arm.[32] The POSITRON trial evaluated 207 patients with GT 2 or 3 infection who were interferon intolerant or ineligible. Subjects were treated with 12 weeks of sofosbuvir and weight-based ribavirin. SVR rates were slightly higher than those reported in the FISSION trial (61.2%). Adverse events were minimal, namely fatigue, insomnia, and anemia, a side effect profile characteristic of ribavirin therapy.[33]

The FUSION trial assessed patients with HCV GT 2 or 3 and history of interferon treatment failure. Patients were treated with sofosbuvir and ribavirin for 12 or 16 weeks. GT 2 SVR rates were 86.1% in the 12-week arm and 93.8% in the 16-week arm. In comparison, lower SVR rates were noted in the GT 3 12- and 16-week treatment arms (29.7% and 61.9%, respectively). The adverse event profile was similar to the one in the POSITRON trial, with no appreciable difference in the 12- and 16-week regimens.[33] Because a longer course increased SVR rates in GT 3 patients, further extension of therapy was evaluated in the VALENCE trial in this population. Sofosbuvir and weight-based ribavirin were administered for 12 weeks in patients with GT 2 infection and 24 weeks in patients with GT 3. In this study, 93% of patients with GT 2 infection achieved SVR. Overall, 85% of patients with GT 3 infection achieved SVR, the highest rate yet.[12] In particular, SVR rates were 95% in treatment-naive patients without cirrhosis and 92% in treatment-naive subjects with cirrhosis. Patients that had failed therapy with pegylated interferon and ribavirin in the past, however, had lower SVR rates (87% in patients without cirrhosis and 62% in patients with cirrhosis). This phase 3 treatment program highlighted the difficulty in eradicating GT 3 infection, particularly in treatment-experienced patients with cirrhosis. In December 2013, the Food and Drug Administration approved a regimen of sofosbuvir and weight-based ribavirin for 24 weeks in GT 3 patients. Although an interferon-free regimen was now available for GT 3, the regimen was suboptimal, with lower SVR rates in treatment-experienced patients with cirrhosis. Furthermore, a 24-week course with ribavirin was required. The impetus to develop new strategies remained.

The BOSON trial involved randomization of HCV GT 3–infected subjects to peginterferon alfa plus sofosbuvir and ribavirin for 12 weeks versus sofosbuvir plus ribavirin for 16 or 24 weeks. Patients who received peginterferon alfa had higher SVR rates (93%) when compared with those who received sofosbuvir and ribavirin (71% for 16 weeks and 84% for 24 weeks, respectively). Among the treatment-experienced cirrhotic cohort, interferon therapy was found to result in an improved SVR rate (86%) versus 47% and 77% for the 16- and 24-week sofosbuvir and ribavirin treatment arms, respectively.[34]

More recently, sofosbuvir plus daclatasvir, an NS5A inhibitor, have also been studied in patients with HCV GT 1, 2, or 3. In patients with GT 3, subjects were randomized to a 4-week lead-in arm with sofosbuvir followed by sofosbuvir plus daclatasvir for 23 weeks versus sofosbuvir plus daclatasvir for 24 weeks versus sofosbuvir, daclatasvir, and ribavirin for 24 weeks. A total of 85% of patients treated with daclatasvir and sofosbuvir alone demonstrated SVR versus 100% treated with sofosbuvir, daclatasvir, and ribavirin.[35] In ALLY 3, treatment-naive or experienced subjects received 12 weeks of therapy with sofosbuvir plus daclatasvir. The overall SVR rate was 89%, in treatment-naive patients 90%, and in treatment-experienced patients 86%. In patients without cirrhosis, a 97% SVR was observed in treatment-naive patients and a 94% SVR in the treatment experienced cohort. Response rates for patients with cirrhosis were lower, however, with SVR rates of 58% for treatment-naive and 69% for treatment-experienced subjects.[36] Adverse events were minimal, with the most common side effects reported being fatigue, headache, and nausea. This 12-week, interferon and ribavirin-free regimen is appealing for GT 3 patients. Data from the ALLY-3+ study were published evaluating the response of daclatasvir in combination with sofosbuvir and ribavirin for 12 or 16 weeks. This study included only GT 3–infected patients with advanced fibrosis or cirrhosis who were either treatment naive or experienced, although patients previously exposed to NS5A inhibitors were excluded. The overall SVR rate was 92% (91% in those treated with 12 weeks and 92% in those treated for 16 weeks). In patients with advanced fibrosis alone, a 100% response rate was observed with both 12 and 16 weeks of therapy. Response rates were slightly lower for patients treated who had underlying cirrhosis (88% with 12 weeks of therapy vs 89% for 16 weeks of therapy). In the treatment-experienced cirrhotic cohort, 12 weeks of therapy yielded an 88% response rate versus an 86% response rate with 16 weeks of therapy. The primary side effects observed were insomnia, headache, and fatigue, although none resulted in treatment discontinuation. Ribavirin dose reduction was undertaken in 12% of patients.[36]

An extended duration of therapy with 24 weeks of daclatasvir and sofosbuvir with or without ribavirin has also been assessed as part of the European Multicenter Compassionate Use Program. This study enrolled patients infected with HCV at risk of decompensation within 12 months. Most of the patients in this study were cirrhotic (91%) with GT 3–infected patients comprising 17% of those studied. Response rates for GT 3–infected patients overall were 92%, with 85% who received sofosbuvir and ribavirin achieving SVR compared with 100% in those who received sofosbuvir, dactlatasivr, plus ribavirin. The most common side effects were headache, nausea, fatigue, and anemia, the latter of which was observed in the ribavirin-containing arms[37]

Ledipasvir, an NS5A inhibitor, has also been studied in GT 3–infected patients in combination with sofosbuvir. The ELECTRON-2 trial assessed response rates of sofosbuvir plus ledipasvir with or without ribavirin for 12 weeks in GT 1– and 3–infected individuals. Response rates of 100% were observed in treatment-naive GT 3 patients receiving ribavirin, although response rates were lower in treatment-naive patients not administered ribavirin (64%).[38] Of note, this study included 15% GT 3–infected patients with cirrhosis, but the response rates for this subpopulation were not reported.

Another treatment recently approved includes sofosbuvir plus velpatasvir, an NS5A inhibitor with pan-genotypic activity. In one study, treatment-naive, GT 3–infected patients without cirrhosis were treated with sofosbuvir and velpatasvir with or without ribavirin for 8 weeks. In this study, patients who received 100 mg of velpatasvir had response rates of 96% without ribavirin and 100% with ribavirin.[39] In a subsequent trial, GT 1– and 3–infected patients, treatment naive or treatment experienced, were administered 12 weeks of sofosbuvir plus velpatasvir with or without ribavirin. This study, which included subjects with cirrhosis, demonstrated response rates of 100% in GT 3–infected patients without cirrhosis with 100 mg of velpatasvir with or without ribavirin. In patients with cirrhosis, 100% response rates were achieved with adjunctive ribavirin compared with SVR rates of 88% without ribavirin.[40]

Data from the ASTRAL-3 trial were published showing favorable response rates for GT 3–infected individuals. In this study, treatment-naive and -experienced patients with GT 3 infection were treated with sofosbuvir and ribavirin for 24 weeks versus sofosbuvir and velpatasvir for 12 weeks. This trial, which included subjects with cirrhosis, demonstrated a 95% response rate in the velpatasvir arm versus 80% in the regimen containing sofosbuvir and ribavirin alone. Side effects were minimal in the velpatasvir-containing arm, consisting primarily of headache and fatigue, with no treatment discontinuations attributed to adverse events.[41] In regard to patients with GT 3 infection and decompensated cirrhosis, the ASTRAL-4 study assessed 12 weeks of velpatasvir and sofosbuvir with or without ribavirin compared with velpatasvir and sofosbuvir alone for 24 weeks. Response rates for 12 weeks of therapy without ribavirin were 50% as compared with 85% for 12 weeks of therapy with ribavirin. For those patients who received 24 weeks of therapy without ribavirin, response rates of 50% were observed.[42] A recent paper assessing patient-related outcomes in individuals with both compensated and decompensated cirrhosis treated with velpatasvir and sofosbuvir found a significant improvement in patient-related outcome scores during treatment and following SVR. These scores were more significant among those patients who had decompensated cirrhosis.[43]

Another study assessed sofosbuvir in conjunction with grazoprevir, an NS3/4A protease inhibitor, and elbasvir, an NS5A inhibitor. Treatment regimens with grazoprevir and elbasvir can be used in patients with renal dysfunction, including those on hemodialysis.[44] Sofosbuvir, however, is not recommended in patients with severe renal insufficiency or who are on dialysis. These agents, when used in treatment-naive GT 3 patients without cirrhosis for either 8 or 12 weeks of therapy, were found to yield response rates of 93% and 100%, respectively. Of those patients who had underlying cirrhosis, response rates were 91% after 12 weeks of treatment.[45]

Emerging Therapies for Genotype 3

Glecaprevir/pibrentasvir

Glecaprevir, an NS3/NS4A inhibitor, and pibrentasvir, an NS5A inhibitor, are two emerging therapies currently being studied. These drugs have minimal renal excretion, thus being a viable option for patients with significant renal dysfunction, including individuals who are on hemodialysis. In the EXPEDITION-IV study, a total of 104 patients with renal insufficiency were treated, 82% of whom were on hemodialysis. In the modified intention-to-treat analysis, 100% of patients achieved SVR 12 after treatment for 12 weeks. Eleven percent of the patients in this study had GT 3 infection, with 19% of the overall cohort having cirrhosis, none of whom were decompensated. No major side effects were observed, with most treatment-related side effects being pruritus (20%), fatigue (14%), and nausea (12%).[46]

Grazoprevir/ruzasvir/uprifosbuvir

Grazoprevir/ruzasvir/uprifosbuvir is a combination of an NS3/NS4 inhibitor (grazoprevir), a new pangenotypic NS5A inhibitor (ruzasvir), and a new NS5B polymerase inhibitor (uprifosbuvir). In Part B of C-CREST-1&2, this combination was studied in patients with HCV GTs 1, 2, or 3 infection. Patients were either treatment naive or treatment experienced with prior interferon-based therapies. Treatment was administered for 8, 12, or 16 weeks, with or without ribavirin. This study included a total of 337 GT 3–infected patients, 35% of whom had cirrhosis. Sustained virologic rates for 8, 12, and 16 weeks of therapy were 95%, 97%, and 96%, respectively. Regarding ribavirin, in the 8-week group, response rates of 94% without ribavirin and 98% with ribavirin were noted. In the 12-week arms, individuals who did not receive ribavirin had response rates of 97% versus 99% with ribavirin. In the 16-week group, numerically higher response rates were found in those who did not receive ribavirin (98%) as compared with those who did (96%). Response rates in patients with compensated cirrhosis were not significantly different, and included SVR rates of 100% at 12 weeks with ribavirin and 100% at 16 weeks without ribavirin. In patients who were both treatment-experienced and had cirrhosis, 100% response rates were achieved at 12 weeks with and without ribavirin and at 16 weeks without ribavirin. Pretreatment RAVs were found in 4% of patients treated for 8 weeks and 5% of those treated for 12 weeks, with response rates in that population of 50% in the 8-week arm and 71% in the 12-week arm. Minor common side effects included headache (22%), fatigue (19%), and nausea (13%), with one death during the study period caused by bacterial sepsis unrelated to study-drug.[47]

In patients who relapsed to a short course (8 weeks) of antiviral therapy with grazoprevir, uprifosbuvir, and either elbasvir or ruzasvir in an earlier trial, C-CREST Part C studied retreatment with grazoprevir, ruzasvir, and uprifosbuvir and ribavirin for 16 weeks. A total of 24 patients were enrolled, eight of whom had GT 3 infection. RAVs to NS3 were found in all eight patients, and seven of eight had NS5A RAVs. All patients with GT 3 infection who were retreated achieved SVR 12. The results of this study are reflective of efficacy of retreatment despite treatment failure when a truncated duration of therapy was used.[48]

The issue of resistance

Testing for RAVs is recommended in patients prone to treatment failure or relapse, particularly those who have cirrhosis, are treatment naive, or both. When detected, they may help to identify patients who may require a longer duration of therapy and/or addition of ribavirin to optimize SVR rates.[9]

Emerging Therapies for Direct-Acting Antiviral Failures

Sofosbuvir/velpatasvir/voxilaprevir

Sofosbuvir, velpatasvir, and voxilaprevir, a new pangenotypic NS3/NS4 inhibitor, have been examined in patients with GT 3. In the POLARIS-1 study, 263 patients who previously were exposed to NS5A inhibitors were treated with a 12-week course of the three medications. Thirty percent had GT 3; 46% of the overall cohort was cirrhotic. SVR 12 was noted in 96% of the overall treatment cohort, and 93% of cirrhotics. SVR rates in patients with GT 3, specifically, were 95%. Adverse events were mild and included headaches (25%), fatigue (21%), diarrhea (18%), and nausea (14%). RAVs were noted in 83% of patients overall, with 79% having NS5A RAVs. A total of 96% of subjects with any RAV achieved SVR 12, and 94% with NS5A RAVs achieved SVR 12. This regimen, which should soon be available, seems to be a viable solution for patients who have failed an NS5A inhibitor.[49]

Whereas POLARIS-1 enrolled patients who were treatment experienced to NS5A inhibitors, POLARIS-4 enrolled patients who were treatment experienced with NS3/4A protease inhibitors and NS5B inhibitors. In this study, patients with GTs 1 to 6 were randomized in a one-to-one fashion to sofosbuvir, velpatasvir, or voxilaprevir versus sofosbuvir and velpatasvir alone for 12 weeks. Forty-six percent of the overall cohort had compensated cirrhosis. Among those with GT 3 infection, 54 were randomized to sofosbuvir, velpatasvir, and voxilaprevir with 94% achieving SVR 12 as compared with 85% of the 52 patients randomized to sofosbuvir and velpatasvir for 12 weeks. Treatment side effects were similar to those seen in POLARIS-1 with no discontinuations related to adverse drug-related events.[50]

Glecaprevir/pibrentasvir

This regimen has been studied in patients with DAA failure. In the SURVEYOR-II, Part 3 trial, 131 GT 3–infected patients were randomized to 12 or 16 weeks of therapy. Patients who were treatment naive or experienced, with or without cirrhosis, were included. RAVs were identified at baseline in 21%, most being NS5A RAVs (18% overall). Treatment-experienced patients without cirrhosis randomized to 12 or 16 weeks of therapy achieved SVR 12 rates of 91% and 96%, respectively. Treatment-naive patients with cirrhosis treated for 12 weeks achieved SVR 12 rates of 98%, and treatment-experienced patients with cirrhosis had response rates of 96%. The most common side effects reported were fatigue and headache, with no treatment discontinuations attributed to study drug. The combination of these two agents, which should soon be available, will provide a viable option for GT 3 patients with prior treatment experience.

CURRENT TREATMENT RECOMMENDATIONS

It should be noted that the landscape for HCV therapy is rapidly changing given the advent of newer DAA therapies. A guidance document with treatment recommendations from the American Association of the Study for Liver Diseases and the Infectious Diseases of America is frequently updated to reflect the changing landscape.

Currently, for treatment-naive GT 3–infected patients without cirrhosis, 12 weeks of daclatasvir plus sofosbuvir are recommended. An alternate recommended regimen for this population is velpatasvir and sofosbuvir for 12 weeks (**Table 1**).

For patients who are treatment naive with cirrhosis, 12 weeks of velpatasvir plus sofosbuvir are recommended. As an alternative regimen, 24 weeks of therapy with daclatasvir plus sofosbuvir with or without weight-based ribavirin is recommended.

In patients who are treatment experienced with interferon and without cirrhosis, 12 weeks of daclatasvir plus sofosbuvir or the combination of velpatasvir plus sofosbuvir for 12 weeks are recommended. For patients who are treatment experienced with cirrhosis, 12 weeks of velpatasvir plus sofosbuvir and weight-based ribavirin or elbasvir/grazoprevir plus sofosbuvir for 12 weeks are recommended. An alternate to these regimens is 24 weeks of daclatasvir plus sofosbuvir with weight-based ribavirin.

In patients who are treatment experienced with a sofosbuvir-containing regimen, who do not require urgent treatment, and who do not have evidence of cirrhosis, treatment deferral is recommended. For those who require urgent treatment regardless of cirrhosis status, 24 weeks of daclatasvir plus sofosbuvir with weight-based ribavirin is recommended. An alternate to this is 12 weeks of velpatasvir and sofosbuvir with weight-based ribavirin.

Table 1
Current American Association of the Study for Liver Diseases treatment recommendations for genotype 3 infection

	Noncirrhotic	Cirrhotic
Treatment naive	DCV + SOF × 12 wk VEL + SOF × 12 wk	DCV + SOF ± R × 24 wk VEL + SOF × 12 wk
Treatment experienced (interferon)	DCV + SOF × 12 wk VEL + SOF × 12 wk	DCV + SOF + R × 24 wk VEL + SOF + R × 12 wk ELB/GRA + SOF × 12 wk

Treatment experienced (sofosbuvir)	Defer therapy (nonurgent)
	If urgent
	  DCV + SOF + R × 24 wk
	  VEL + SOF + R × 12 wk
	  ELB/GRA + SOF × 12 wk
		DCV + SOF + R × 24 wk
		VEL + SOF + R × 12 wk
		ELB/GRA + SOF × 12 wk

	Decompensated cirrhosis	LDV + SOF + r × 24 wk DCV + SOF + r × 24 wk VEL + SOF + R × 12 wk

Abbreviations: DCV, daclatasvir; ELB/GRA, elbasvir/grazoprevir; SOF, sofosbuvir; SOF + r, sofosbuvir with low-dose ribavirin; SOF + R, sofosbuvir with weight-based ribavirin; VEL, velpatasvir.

Table 2
Treatment response rates by regimen

	Treatment-Naive Noncirrhotic, %	Treatment-Experienced Noncirrhotic, %	Treatment-Naive Cirrhotic, %	Treatment-Experienced Cirrhotic, %
SOF + R × 24 wk (VALENCE)	95	92	87	62
SOF + PR × 12 wk (BOSON)	96	91	94	86
SOF + DCV × 12 wk (ALLY-3)	97	94	58	69
	Overall	Noncirrhotic	Overall	Cirrhotic
SOF + DCV × 24 wk		N/A		100
	Treatment	Naive	Treatment	Experienced
SOF + LDV + R × 12 wk (ELECTRON-2)		100		82
	Treatment-naive noncirrhotic	Treatment-naive cirrhotic	Treatment-experienced noncirrhotic	Treatment-experienced cirrhotic
SOF + VEL × 12 wk (ASTRAL -3)	98	93	91	89
	Treatment-naive noncirrhotic 8 wk	Treatment-naive noncirrhotic 12 wk		Treatment-naive cirrhotic 12 wk
SOF + ELB/GRA × 8–12 wk	100	100		91

Abbreviations: DCV, daclatasvir; ELB, elbasvir; GRA, grazoprevir; LDV, ledipasvir; PR, Peg interferon + ribavirin; SOF, sofosbuvir; SOF + R, sofosbuvir with weight-based ribavirin; VEL, velpatasvir.

In individuals with decompensated cirrhosis, ledipasvir with sofosbuvir, and ribavirin (600 mg daily), or daclatasvir with sofosbuvir and ribavirin (600 mg) are recommended for 12 weeks. Ribavirin dosage should be increased as tolerated. An alternate is velpatasvir plus sofosbuvir and weight-based ribavirin for 12 weeks[51]

SUMMARY

GT 3 HCV is associated with a more aggressive clinical course when compared with other HCV GTs. This provides the impetus to actively treat patients with GT 3. Unfortunately, GT 3 has proven to be the most difficult to eradicate with the new DAAs.[6] In particular, treatment-naive and treatment-experienced patients with cirrhosis have the lowest response rates. With the current regimens, it seems that longer courses and the addition of ribavirin may improve response rates (**Table 2**). Effective, well-tolerated regimens are now available. For patients who have failed therapy with DAAs, new regimens should be available in the near future. Antiviral therapy for patients with GT 3 should be implemented when possible.

REFERENCES

1. Davis GL, Alter MJ, El-Serag H, et al. Aging of hepatitis C virus (HCV)-infected persons in the United States: a multiple cohort model of HCV prevalence and disease progression. Gastroenterology 2010;138(2):513–21, 521.e1-6.
2. Planas R, Balleste B, Alvarez MA, et al. Natural history of decompensated hepatitis C virus-related cirrhosis. A study of 200 patients. J Hepatol 2004;40(5):823–30.
3. Coilly A, Roche B, Duclos-Vallee JC, et al. Management of post transplant hepatitis C in the direct antiviral agents era. Hepatol Int 2015;9(2):192–201.
4. Ghany MG, Nelson DR, Strader DB, et al, American Association for Study of Liver Diseases. An update on treatment of genotype 1 chronic hepatitis C virus infection: 2011 practice guideline by the American Association for the Study of Liver Diseases. Hepatology 2011;54(4):1433–44.
5. Muir AJ, Naggie S. Hepatitis C virus treatment: is it possible to cure all hepatitis C virus patients? Clin Gastroenterol Hepatol 2015;13(12):2166–72.
6. Tapper EB, Afdhal NH. Is 3 the new 1: perspectives on virology, natural history and treatment for hepatitis C genotype 3. J Viral Hepat 2013;20(10):669–77.
7. Nkontchou G, Ziol M, Aout M, et al. HCV genotype 3 is associated with a higher hepatocellular carcinoma incidence in patients with ongoing viral C cirrhosis. J Viral Hepat 2011;18(10):e516–22.
8. McCombs J, Matsuda T, Tonnu-Mihara I, et al. The risk of long-term morbidity and mortality in patients with chronic hepatitis C: results from an analysis of data from a Department of Veterans Affairs Clinical Registry. JAMA Intern Med 2014;174(2):204–12.
9. Zeuzem S, Mizokami M, Pianko S, et al. NS5A resistance-associated substitutions in patients with genotype 1 hepatitis C virus: prevalence and effect on treatment outcome. J Hepatol 2017;66(5):910–8.
10. Messina JP, Humphreys I, Flaxman A, et al. Global distribution and prevalence of hepatitis C virus genotypes. Hepatology 2015;61(1):77–87.
11. Gower E, Estes C, Blach S, et al. Global epidemiology and genotype distribution of the hepatitis C virus infection. J Hepatol 2014;61(1 Suppl):S45–57.
12. Zeuzem S, Dusheiko GM, Salupere R, et al. Sofosbuvir and ribavirin in HCV genotypes 2 and 3. N Engl J Med 2014;370(21):1993–2001.

13. Arrese M, Riquelme A, Soza A. Insulin resistance, hepatic steatosis and hepatitis C: a complex relationship with relevant clinical implications. Ann Hepatol 2010; 9(Suppl):112–8.
14. Castera L, Hezode C, Roudot-Thoraval F, et al. Effect of antiviral treatment on evolution of liver steatosis in patients with chronic hepatitis C: indirect evidence of a role of hepatitis C virus genotype 3 in steatosis. Gut 2004;53(3):420–4.
15. Poynard T, Ratziu V, McHutchison J, et al. Effect of treatment with peginterferon or interferon alfa-2b and ribavirin on steatosis in patients infected with hepatitis C. Hepatology 2003;38(1):75–85.
16. Asselah T, Boyer N, Guimont MC, et al. Liver fibrosis is not associated with steatosis but with necroinflammation in French patients with chronic hepatitis C. Gut 2003;52(11):1638–43.
17. Rubbia-Brandt L, Fabris P, Paganin S, et al. Steatosis affects chronic hepatitis C progression in a genotype specific way. Gut 2004;53(3):406–12.
18. Abid K, Pazienza V, de Gottardi A, et al. An in vitro model of hepatitis C virus genotype 3a-associated triglycerides accumulation. J Hepatol 2005;42(5):744–51.
19. Roingeard P. Hepatitis C virus diversity and hepatic steatosis. J Viral Hepat 2013; 20(2):77–84.
20. Bochud PY, Cai T, Overbeck K, et al. Genotype 3 is associated with accelerated fibrosis progression in chronic hepatitis C. J Hepatol 2009;51(4):655–66.
21. Adinolfi LE, Gambardella M, Andreana A, et al. Steatosis accelerates the progression of liver damage of chronic hepatitis C patients and correlates with specific HCV genotype and visceral obesity. Hepatology 2001;33(6):1358–64.
22. Kumar D, Farrell GC, Fung C, et al. Hepatitis C virus genotype 3 is cytopathic to hepatocytes: reversal of hepatic steatosis after sustained therapeutic response. Hepatology 2002;36(5):1266–72.
23. Rubbia-Brandt L, Quadri R, Abid K, et al. Hepatocyte steatosis is a cytopathic effect of hepatitis C virus genotype 3. J Hepatol 2000;33(1):106–15.
24. Kanwal F, Kramer JR, Ilyas J, et al. HCV genotype 3 is associated with an increased risk of cirrhosis and hepatocellular cancer in a national sample of U.S. Veterans with HCV. Hepatology 2014;60(1):98–105.
25. Ghany MG, Strader DB, Thomas DL, et al. Diseases AAftSoL. Diagnosis, management, and treatment of hepatitis C: an update. Hepatology 2009;49(4): 1335–74.
26. European Association for the Study of the Liver. EASL Clinical Practice Guidelines: management of hepatitis C virus infection. J Hepatol 2011;55(2):245–64.
27. Fried MW, Shiffman ML, Reddy KR, et al. Peginterferon alfa-2a plus ribavirin for chronic hepatitis C virus infection. N Engl J Med 2002;347(13):975–82.
28. Hadziyannis SJ, Sette H Jr, Morgan TR, et al. Peginterferon-alpha2a and ribavirin combination therapy in chronic hepatitis C: a randomized study of treatment duration and ribavirin dose. Ann Intern Med 2004;140(5):346–55.
29. Manns MP, McHutchison JG, Gordon SC, et al. Peginterferon alfa-2b plus ribavirin compared with interferon alfa-2b plus ribavirin for initial treatment of chronic hepatitis C: a randomised trial. Lancet 2001;358(9286):958–65.
30. Zeuzem S, Hultcrantz R, Bourliere M, et al. Peginterferon alfa-2b plus ribavirin for treatment of chronic hepatitis C in previously untreated patients infected with HCV genotypes 2 or 3. J Hepatol 2004;40(6):993–9.
31. Mangia A, Santoro R, Minerva N, et al. Peginterferon alfa-2b and ribavirin for 12 vs. 24 weeks in HCV genotype 2 or 3. N Engl J Med 2005;352(25):2609–17.
32. Lawitz E, Mangia A, Wyles D, et al. Sofosbuvir for previously untreated chronic hepatitis C infection. N Engl J Med 2013;368(20):1878–87.

33. Jacobson IM, Gordon SC, Kowdley KV, et al. Sofosbuvir for hepatitis C genotype 2 or 3 in patients without treatment options. N Engl J Med 2013;368(20):1867–77.

34. Foster GR, Pianko S, Cooper C, et al. Sofosbuvir plus Peg-IFN/RBV for 12 weeks versus sofosbuvir/RBV for 16 or 24 weeks in genotype 3 HCV-infected patients and treatment-experienced cirrhotic patients with genotype 2 HCV: the BOSON Study. Abstract 2015; Program and abstracts of the 50th Annual Meeting of the European Association for the Study of the Liver. Vienna, Austria, April 22–26, 2015.

35. Sulkowski MS, Jacobson IM, Nelson DR. Daclatasvir plus sofosbuvir for HCV infection. N Engl J Med 2014;370(16):1560–1.

36. Nelson DR, Cooper JN, Lalezari JP, et al. All-oral 12-week treatment with daclatasvir plus sofosbuvir in patients with hepatitis C virus genotype 3 infection: ALLY-3 phase III study. Hepatology 2015;61(4):1127–35.

37. Welzel TM, Herzer K, Ferenci P, et al. Daclatasvir plus sofosbuvir with or without ribavirin for the treatment of HCV in patients with severe liver disease: interim results of a multicenter compassionate use program. Vienna, Austria, EASL April 22–26, Abstract 2015.

38. Gane EJ, Hyland RH, An D. Sofosbuvir/ledipasvir fixed dose combination is safe and effective in difficult-to-treat populations including genotype-3 patients, decompensated genotype-1 patients, and genotype-1 patients with prior sofosbuvir treatment experience. Abstract 2014; Program and abstracts of the 49th Annual Meeting of the European Association for the Study of the Liver. London, England, April 9–13, 2014.

39. Gane EJ, Hyland RH, An, D, et al. Once-daily sofosbuvir with GS-5816 for 8 weeks with or without ribavirin in patients with HCV genotype 3 without cirrhosis result in high rates of SVR12: the ELECTRON-2 Study. Abstract AASLD 2014 Boston, November 8–11, 2014.

40. Pianko S, Flamm SL, Shiffman ML, et al. Sofosbuvir plus velpatasvir combination therapy for treatment-experienced patients with genotype 1 or 3 hepatitis C virus infection: a randomized trial. Ann Intern Med 2015;163(11):809–17.

41. Foster GR, Afdhal N, Roberts SK, et al. Sofosbuvir and velpatasvir for HCV genotype 2 and 3 infection. N Engl J Med 2015;373(27):2608–17.

42. Curry MP, O'Leary JG, Bzowej N, et al. Sofosbuvir and velpatasvir for HCV in patients with decompensated cirrhosis. N Engl J Med 2015;373(27):2618–28.

43. Younossi ZM, Stepanova M, Feld J, et al. Sofosbuvir and velpatasvir combination improves patient-reported outcomes for patients with HCV infection, without or with compensated or decompensated cirrhosis. Clin Gastroenterol Hepatol 2017;15(3):421–30.e6.

44. Roth D, Nelson DR, Bruchfeld A, et al. Grazoprevir plus elbasvir in treatment-naive and treatment-experienced patients with hepatitis C virus genotype 1 infection and stage 4-5 chronic kidney disease (the C-SURFER study): a combination phase 3 study. Lancet 2015;386(10003):1537–45.

45. Lawitz E, Poordad F, Gutierrez JA, et al. Short-duration treatment with elbasvir/grazoprevir and sofosbuvir for hepatitis C: a randomized trial. Hepatology 2017;65(2):439–50.

46. Gane E. EXPEDITION-IV: Safety and efficacy of GLE/PIB in adults with renal impairment and chronic hepatitis C virus genotype 1-6 infection. 67th Annual Meeting of the American Association for the Study of Liver Diseases. Boston, USA, November 11–15, abstract LB-11, 2016.

47. Lawitz E. Safety and efficacy of the fixed-dose combination regimen of MK-3682/grazoprevir/MK-8408 (ruzasvir) with or without ribavirin in non-cirrhotic or cirrhotic

patients with chronic HCV GT1, 2 or 3 infection (Part B of C-CREST-1 & -2) Presented at the American Association for the Study of Liver Disease. Boston, MA, November 11–15, 2016.

48. Serfaty EA. High sustained virologic response rates in patients with chronic HCV GT1, 2 or 3 infection following 16 weeks of MK-3682, grazoprevir/MK-8408 (ruzasvir) plus ribavirin after failure of 8 weeks of therapy (Part C of C-CREST-1 &2) Presented at the American Association for the Study of Liver Disease. Boston, MA, November 7–11, 2016.

49. Bourlière MEA. Sofosbuvir/velpatasvir/voxilaprevir for 12 weeks as a salvage regimen in NS5A inhibitor-experienced patients with genotype 1-6 infection: the phase 3 POLARIS-1 Study, presented at the American Association for the Study of Liver Diseases Meeting. Boston, MA, November 7–11, 2016.

50. Zeuzem S. A randomized, controlled, phase 3 trial of sofosbuvir/velpatasvir/voxilaprevir or sofosbuvir/velpatasvir for 12 weeks in direct-acting antiviral-experienced patients with genotype 1-6 HCV infection: the POLARIS-4 Study Presented at the American Association of the Study of Liver Disease. Boston, MA, November, 2016.

51. Recommendations for testing, managing, and treating hepatitis C. Joint panel from the American Association of the Study of Liver Diseases and the Infectious Diseases Society of America. 2014. Available at: http://www.hcvguidelines.org/. Accessed October 6, 2015.

Primer on Hepatitis C Virus Resistance to Direct-Acting Antiviral Treatment

A Practical Approach for the Treating Physician

Ilan S. Weisberg, MD*, Ira M. Jacobson, MD

KEYWORDS

- Hepatitis C virus (HCV) • Direct-acting antiviral (DAA)
- Resistance-associated substitution (RAS)

KEY POINTS

- Interferon-free DAA regimens have vastly transformed the HCV landscape and the promise of cure is within reach for all patients living with chronic HCV infection.
- Combinations of inhibitors already have the power to cure more than 90% of patients and additional combinations of next-generation DAAs are just around the corner.
- The role of RAS testing is slowly emerging; these substitutions clearly have a negative impact on the chance of cure in specific HCV populations, particularly genotype 1a and 3 patients with prior treatment failure and advanced liver disease, and in these settings pretreatment RAS testing and modification of treatment is appropriate.
- Because the effect of these RASs can seemingly be abrogated by extending or intensifying treatment, it is possible that any degree of HCV resistance could be overcome with longer duration or more potent treatments.

INTRODUCTION

Hepatitis C virus (HCV) infects more than 170 million people worldwide and is a leading cause of progressive liver damage, cirrhosis, and hepatocellular carcinoma. Curative therapies historically relied on interferon-based treatments and were limited by significant toxicity and poor response rates, particularly among patients with prior treatment failure and advanced hepatic fibrosis. The recent advent of direct-acting antivirals (DAA) agents targeting key steps in the HCV viral life cycle has transformed the

Disclosure: I.S. Weisberg has received a Speaker's honorarium from Gilead, Merck, and Intercept. I.M. Jacobson is a Consultant for Bristol-Myers Squibb, Gilead, Intercept, Janssen, Merck, and Trek; and has received a Speaker's honorarium from Gilead, Intercept, and Merck.
Division of Digestive Diseases, Mount Sinai Beth Israel Medical Center, Icahn School of Medicine at Mount Sinai, 10 Union Square East, Suite 2G, New York, NY 10003, USA
* Corresponding author.
E-mail address: ilan.weisberg@mountsinai.org

Clin Liver Dis 21 (2017) 659–672
http://dx.doi.org/10.1016/j.cld.2017.06.007
1089-3261/17/© 2017 Elsevier Inc. All rights reserved.

liver.theclinics.com

landscape of HCV treatment by offering highly effective and well-tolerated interferon-free, DAA-based combination therapies. However, depending on the characteristics of the patients being treated, the selected treatment regimen, and the susceptibility of the virus, a small proportion of patients fail to be cured with currently approved DAA regimens.[1–3] The emergence of viral resistance to a DAA, especially in the NS5A inhibitor drug class, during the course of antiviral therapy is the most common cause of DAA failure. This clinical review serves as a primer on HCV resistance to DAA therapy and is intended for the treating clinician. We review the principles of HCV resistance, the impact that pre-existing resistance to current DAA regimens plays in virologic failure, and the role of resistance testing before initial treatment and after treatment failure (**Table 1**).

HEPATITIS C VIRUS: GENETIC VARIABILITY

HCV is a member of the Flaviviridae virus family.[4] It consists of a single-stranded RNA genome approximately 9600 nucleotides in length that encodes a large polyprotein that contains three structural (core, E1, and E2) and seven nonstructural proteins (p7, NS2, NS3, NS4A, NS4B, NS5A, and NS5B). Short untranslated regions at each end of the genome are required for translation and replication.[4] The high replication rate of the virus, coupled with the high error rate of its RNA-dependent RNA polymerase, has allowed the HCV virus to evolve with tremendous global diversity. At present time, seven distinct genetic lineages exist and account for the seven known HCV genotypes (1 through 7) and 67 subtypes.[5] The genomes of the seven different genotypes differ from each other by at least 30% at the nucleotide level, and the subtypes within a given genotype differ between 15% and 25%.[5] In Western countries, subtypes 1a, 1b, and 3a account for most chronic infections.

In addition to the different genotypes and subtypes, HCV diversity continues at the nucleotide level. The error-prone HCV RNA polymerase lacks a proofreading mechanism and generates an estimated 10^{-4} substitutions per round of replication.[6] The high rate of error, coupled with the rapid rate of replication, continually generates large numbers of genetically distinct, but closely related, viral variants during chronic infection. As such, patients are infected with a complex mixture of viral populations, whose relative proportions depend on their replication capacities (also known as fitness). This cloud of viral variants is termed the quasispecies[2,4,7,8] and is central to understanding

Table 1		
DAAs currently approved for the treatment of chronic HCV infection		
Class	**Compound**	**Manufacturer**
NS5B polymerase inhibitor	Sofosbuvir (nucleotide analogue)	Gilead
	Dasabuvir (nonnucleotide inhibitor)	AbbVie
NS5A protein inhibitor	Daclatasvir	Bristol-Myers Squibb
	Ledipasvir	Gilead
	Ombitasvir	AbbVie
	Elbasvir	Merck
	Velpatasvir	Gilead
NS3-4A protease inhibitor	Simeprevir	Janssen
	Paritaprevir/r[a]	AbbVie
	Asunaprevir	Bristol-Myers Squibb
	Grazoprevir	Merck

[a] Ritonavir boosted.

the dynamics of DAA resistance and the possibility for virologic failure because the genetic diversity it achieves creates the potential to rapidly adapt to a changing environment.[2]

Naturally occurring mutations that arise in viral proteins critical for the antiviral effect of a DAA may confer reduced susceptibility to a specific DAA or an entire DAA class. These mutations can arise in any of the key targets of DAA treatment including the NS3 protease, the NS5B polymerase, and the NS5A protein[9,10] and are typically associated with a change in the conformation of the binding site of the DAA to the target HCV protein. Such mutations do arise spontaneously but are often deleterious and result in reduced fitness compared with the wild-type virus. As such, they typically represent minor viral populations within the quasispecies. However, when a DAA is administered and wild-type virus is inhibited, these low-fitness, DAA-resistant minor variants undergo positive selection and can rapidly outpace the wild-type strain leading to viral resistance.[9] This example illustrates an important concept of a quasispecies infection; the quasispecies as a whole, rather than a particular variant, is the target of a particular selection process or antiviral regimen.[4]

The impact that a given resistance-associated substitution (RAS) has on the antiviral activity of a DAA agent is highly variable. In vitro, the magnitude of resistance conferred by a given RAS is assessed using the HCV replicon system. Individual point mutations are introduced into the viral genome and the 50% inhibitory concentration (IC_{50}), defined as the concentration of the drug required for 50% inhibition, is determined for each DAA-RAS pair and expressed as a fold-change compared with the wild-type replicon. IC_{50} and 50% effective concentration (EC_{50}) are often used interchangeably, although EC_{50} more accurately describes the plasma concentration required for achieving 50% of a maximum effect in vivo. Assays that assess the overall sensitivity of an individual's entire quasispecies to specific DAAs are being developed.[11,12]

NOMENCLATURE OF RESISTANCE

During the days of interferon-based HCV treatment, antiviral resistance was not generally a concern. However, with the arrival of interferon-free DAA-based treatment, the potential impact of pre-existing mutations and those emerging during treatment must be considered. Within the literature on this topic, there is substantial variation in the way HCV resistance is described. Recently, a consensus on the preferred terminology for discussing HCV resistance has been achieved.[13] The correct term for any amino acid substitution that confers resistance to an antiviral medication is termed a RAS and the viral variants that contain these RASs are called resistant variants.[2,13] In the past, many authors have used the designation resistance-associated variant in place of RAS, but this term is no longer considered correct, has been removed from the vernacular, and should not be used. By convention, a RAS is reported by its amino acid change in the viral protein. For example, S282T implies that the serine amino acid found in the wild-type virus at position 282 has been replaced with a threonine residue.

RASs are categorized as either drug-specific or class-specific. A class-specific RAS is a substitution that results in reduced susceptibility to any approved or investigational DAA in that DAA class, whereas a drug-specific RAS is one that confers reduced susceptibility to a specific agent alone. RASs are further classified based on the magnitude with which they restrict the antiviral agent. A RAS is considered to be clinically significant if in the in vitro replicon system it is shown to confer at least a two- to five-fold increase in the EC_{50} compared with wild-type virus or if it emerges during the course of DAA treatment.[2] A given RAS may be considered to result in high-level resistance if the EC_{50} change is substantially higher than the cutoff for clinical significance, often reaching effects of greater than 25-fold or even greater than 100-fold compared with the wild-type replicon. Conversely, polymorphic changes at RAS positions may arise that do not impact EC_{50} at all and are therefore not considered clinically relevant.[2,13]

PREVALENCE OF BASELINE RESISTANCE-ASSOCIATED SUBSTITUTIONS BEFORE ANTIVIRAL TREATMENT

The prevalence of naturally occurring RASs in individuals with chronic HCV infection differs by HCV genotype, subtype, and geographic region. Moreover, the prevalence of a given RAS depends on the sensitivity of the assay used because a pre-existing RAS can only be detected if it is above the cutoff of the sequencing method being used. Many RASs may be present below this threshold and therefore be pre-existing but undetectable. The clinical significance of naturally occurring RASs at low frequencies within the quasispecies is not clear.

Population-based sequencing is the least sensitive and can identify viral populations only if they represent approximately 15% of the patient's viral population (the precise number may vary in different reports). Deep sequencing (sometimes also called next-generation sequencing) is significantly more sensitive and can identify variants represented in smaller proportions, typically 0.5% to 1% of the quasispecies.[2,14,15] However, the identification of all variants found at low frequencies within the quasispecies may not be essential or even appropriate because it does not seem that naturally occurring viral variants present in low proportions (<15% of the quasispecies) significantly influence response to DAA therapy.[2,3] A RAS cutoff of 15%, on the order of what is identified with population-based sequencing, has been shown in clinical trials to be a better predictor of treatment failure because of selection of resistance variants.[2,3] Therefore, the current consensus is that the 15% cutoff should be used in future clinical trials and clinical practice. Commercially available HCV resistance testing assays use population-based sequencing and only those variants found in approximately 15% or more of the quasispecies are generally reported. Most of the available data are for patients with genotype 1, particularly subtype 1a infection.

NS3-4A Protease Inhibitors

The NS3/4A viral protease cleaves the HCV polyprotein, generating the NS3, NS4A, NS4B, NS5A, and NS5B nonstructural proteins. HCV protease inhibitors (PIs) prevent viral polyprotein cleavage by interacting with the protease substrate binding site. There have been a total of five PIs approved for the treatment of chronic HCV, although only three (simeprevir, paritaprevir, and grazoprevir [GZR]) remain available for use. Data from first-generation PIs (telaprevir and boceprevir) laid the foundation for the understanding about DAA and resistance; however, these earlier agents have been replaced by once-daily, better tolerated PIs and are no longer being manufactured.

Because only a few specific interactions are needed to achieve tight binding of the protease to its substrate the genetic barrier to PI resistance is low and cross-resistance between the various PIs is prevalent.[16,17] However, when RASs arise in the NS3/4A gene they generally result in a significant reduction in viral fitness. This explains why these RASs are infrequent before antiviral therapy and are rapidly replaced by wild-type virus when the selective pressure of PI exposure is lifted.

The frequency of most naturally occurring RASs in the NS3/4A PI protein ranges from 0.1% to 3.1% for patients with genotype 1 infection.[18–20] The only notable exception is Q80K, which is not associated with a significant loss of replicative fitness and, when present, confers high-level resistance to most approved PIs. Using population sequencing with a 15% sensitivity cutoff, 2007 patients with genotype 1 infection were assessed for the presence of pretreatment RAS.[20] Q80K was present in 13.7% overall (274 of 2007), but almost all instances occurred in patients with subtype 1a infection. Among genotype 1a individuals, 29.5% (269 of 911) had the Q80K substitution compared with only 0.5% (5 of 1096) of those with 1b infection.[20] Additionally, substantial global variation in the prevalence of the Q80K RAS has been observed. In North American patients, nearly half (48%) of GT1a patients have Q80K, whereas in South America and Europe the prevalence is much lower, 9% and 19%, respectively.[13,21–24] The observation that the Q80K substitution is associated with reduced sensitivity to the PI simeprevir led to the first-ever recommendation for HCV resistance testing in patients with GT1a infection being recommended for treatment with simprevir, peginterferon, and ribavin,[1] with avoidance of the regimen advised in genotype 1a patients testing positive for Q80K.

NS5B Polymerase Inhibitors

Presently there are only two approved agents that inhibit the NS5B viral RNA polymerase. Sofosbuvir (SOF) is a pangenotypic nucleotide inhibitor with a high barrier to resistance. It acts as a defective substrate and inhibits viral RNA synthesis at the active site of the polymerase through chain termination. In vitro, the signature resistance mutation selected after SOF exposure is S282T. This RAS is associated with a marked reduction in replicative fitness and to date has never been identified before antiviral therapy in any patient, even with deep sequencing assays using a cutoff of 1%.[2,18,25–27] In patients who relapsed after SOF-based therapy, S282T has been occasionally identified, but because of its poor fitness, reversion to wild-type within a few weeks of treatment withdrawal was reported.[26,28] Other substitutions in the NS5B gene identified after SOF-based treatment failure include L159F and V321A; however, these mutations do not confer resistance to SOF in the in vitro replicon assays and their clinical significance is uncertain.[29]

Dasabuvir is a nonnucleoside inhibitor that targets the Palm I domain of the HCV RNA polymerase. It induces a conformational change in the NS5B protein, which in turn impedes viral replication. Binding outside the polymerase active site is a major limitation because it increases the potential for resistance. In addition, because the drug's target site is poorly preserved across genotypes, dasabuvir is only effective in genotype 1a and 1b infection, and is used only in combination with paritaprevir (with low-dose ritonavir boosting) and ombitasvir. Unlike SOF, naturally occurring RASs to dasabuvir are seen. The two most prevalent are C316N and S556G, both of which are associated with low-level resistance.[18,19,30] C316N is unique to genotype 1b, and in these patients has a baseline observed prevalence of 10.9% to 35.6%. S556G is found in up to 6% of patients with genotype 1a and up to 25% of those with 1b.[2,13,30,31] There are limited data on the persistence of these viral variants that emerge after treatment,[30] but preliminary data suggest that they can persist for up to a year or more and they may be more likely to persist when they occur together with NS5A RASs.[31]

NS5A Inhibitors

The NS5A protein plays a central role in regulating HCV replication and host cell interactions and is an essential component of the viral replication complex. This protein is an important target to include in DAA combination treatments. Indeed, nearly all patients currently treated receive an NS5A inhibitor-containing regimen. Presently there are five approved NS5A inhibitors (daclatasvir, ledipasvir [LDV], ombitasvir, elbasvir [EBR], and velpatasvir [VEL]) that inhibit the NS5A replication complex by mechanisms that remain unclear. Novel pangenotypic NS5A inhibitors with broad resistance coverage are in late phases of development or pending approval.

Baseline NS5A RASs are identified in treatment-naive patients,[2,3] most commonly at reference amino acid positions K24, M28, Q30, L31, and Y93. Recently, the prevalence of NS5A class RASs was assessed in more than 5000 individuals from phase 2 and 3 clinical trials.[3] Using the 15% cutoff, at least one NS5A RASs was observed in 13% and 17.6% of patients with GT1a and GT1b infection, respectively. Individual RASs were typically noted to occur at a rate of about 1% to 3% with two important exceptions. The M28V substitution, which confers low- to medium-level resistance, was found in 5.4% of GT1a cases; and the Y93H substitution, which confers medium- to high-level resistance, was found in 10.6% of cases with GT1b. Overall, there were no major geographic differences in the distribution of NS5A RASs in this study.[3]

Unlike substitutions that arise in the viral protease and polymerase, several RASs in the NS5A gene do not have as substantial a negative impact on viral fitness; therefore, they are predicted to persist long after selective pressure is released. This is observed in clinical practice; long-term studies demonstrate persistence of NS5A RASs up to 2 years after treatment failure in most patients.[31,32]

IMPACT OF BASELINE RESISTANCE-ASSOCIATED SUBSTITUTIONS ON TREATMENT OUTCOME

Current interferon-free treatment regimens are highly effective and offer curative therapy to most treated patients. Combinations of antiviral agents that target multiple steps in the viral life cycle and contain nonoverlapping resistance profiles result in sustained virologic response (SVR) in 95% or more of patients treated with these medications. Still, small numbers of patients fail therapy and the role of baseline RASs in virologic failure has been revealed. Recent data suggest that in specific patient groups, such as those with prior treatment experience, advanced liver disease, or specific viral genotype/subtype, those substitutions conferring medium- to high-level resistance may affect treatment outcome when represented in large proportions of the quasispecies (>15%) before DAA therapy. In this section, the observed impact of baseline RASs with the four most commonly used DAA regimens is reviewed.

Ledipasvir/Sofosbuvir

The combination single-tablet regimen (STR) of LDV/SOF is approved for the treatment of chronic HCV with genotype 1, 4, 5, or 6 infection. In the three phase 3 studies (ION-1, ION-2, and ION-3) and the phase 2 Lonestar Study, treatment-naive and experienced genotype 1 patients with and without compensated cirrhosis achieved SVR rates of 94% to 99% with 8, 12, or 24 weeks of LDV/SOF ± ribavirin (RBV).[33–36] At the present time, no formal recommendation exists for baseline RAS testing before using this regimen; however, there is evidence that pre-existing NS5A substitutions could impact chance of cure in certain situations, particularly patients with prior treatment failure, advanced liver disease, and GT1a infection.[3,13]

With SVR rates in this range few patients in each study had virologic failure, making it difficult to discern the impact of pretreatment RAS on treatment outcome. Recently, a pooled analysis of the entire phase 2/3 LDV/SOF development program (n = 2144) was performed to determine the baseline prevalence and effect of NS5A, NS5B, or NS3 substitutions.[13] Overall, the impact was small. For genotype 1b patients, baseline NS5A RASs did not diminish the chance of cure, whereas for genotype 1a patients the impact was small. In treatment-naive genotype 1a patients, pretreatment NS5A RASs that conferred a 100-fold increase in the LDV EC_{50} lead to a reduced SVR when treatment was given for 8 weeks but this negative impact was not seen when treatment was 12 weeks. In treatment-experienced patients, with and without cirrhosis, these high-level resistance mutations were associated with reduced rates of SVR after 12 weeks of LDV/SOF but not when therapy was lengthened to 24 weeks or when LDV/SOF was administered for 12 weeks with RBV. The implication from these findings is that the overall impact of baseline NS5A RASs is minimal and is mitigated by extending treatment or intensifying it by adding an additional agent, such as RBV.[13]

In a partially overlapping study to the one just cited, Zeuzem and colleagues[3] recently reported the effect of pretreatment RASs (15% cutoff) on SVR in 1765 patients treated with an approved LDV/SOF regimen. In treatment-naive GT1b patients, baseline NS5A class and LDV-specific RASs did not impact SVR rates, which ranged from 98% to 99%. Similarly, no difference in SVR was observed in treatment-naive GT1a patients with and without NS5A class RASs (97% vs 98%). However, when analysis was restricted to LDV-specific RASs a small difference was noted (91% vs 99%), which was even more pronounced for high-level LDV-specific RASs with greater than 100-fold change in EC_{50} (88% vs 99%).[3] The greatest impact of pretreatment LDV-specific RASs was seen in GT1a treatment-experienced patients in whom 76% with pretreatment RASs and 97% without achieved an SVR. Nonetheless, at present time there is no formal recommendation for pretreatment RAS testing with this regimen and neither the product package insert nor current society treatment guidelines testing for or modifying treatment when RASs are identified.

Ombitasvir/Paritaprevir/Ritonavir with Dasabuvir

Triple therapy targeting the NS3/4, NS5A, and NS5B with ritonavir-boosted paritaprevir, ombitasvir, and dasabuvir (PrOD) with and without RBV was studied in more than 2500 patients in two phase 2 studies (M13–386, AVIATOR) and six phase 3 studies (SAPHIRE-I and –II; PEARL-II, -III, -IV; and TURQUOISE-II).[37–40] In this large clinical trial program only 74 patients experienced a virologic failure, 67 (91%) with GT1a and 7 (9%) with GT1b infection.[30,31,41]

In the phase 2 AVIATOR study, the overall rate of SVR was not affected by the presence or absence of baseline RASs (91% vs 91%),[41] although subanalysis in GT1a patients showed a possible effect. All GT1b patients achieved SVR. Among GT1a patients, 86% (19 of 22) with baseline RASs achieved and SVR compared with 92% (185 of 201) of those without.[41]

To better assess the impact of baseline RASs in each of the three target proteins, population sequencing was performed for the NS3, NS5A, and NS5B regions in a subset of 700 treated GT1a and 1b patients[41] from the entire phase 2 and 3 clinical program. As anticipated, baseline RASs in NS3 were rare (<1%) for GT1a and 1b patients. By comparison, pretreatment RASs were commonly observed in NS5A (12.5% of GT1a and 7.5% of GT1b) and NS5B (5.2% of GT1a and 28.6% of GT1b). A total of 0.4% and 3% of GT1a and 1b patients had baseline RASs in two target proteins, although no individuals had substitutions in all three. Overall, no difference in treatment outcome was observed among those with and without baseline RASs.[41] It should be noted that this three-drug regimen is already designed in such a way as to cover the possibility of NS5A RASs because the use of RBV is stipulated for all genotype 1a patients who receive this regimen. Indeed, the mechanism by which RBV, a weak antiviral against HCV in its own right, exerts a role when combined with far more powerful antiviral agents seems to be by helping to control the emergence of resistant variants.

Recently, in keeping with the previously mentioned conclusion, the effect of baseline RASs restricted to label-recommended dosing of PrOD ± RBV was pooled from four phase 3 trials and reported.[42] Noncirrhotic GT1a-infected patients treated with PrOD + RBV for 12 weeks and those with compensated cirrhosis treated for 24 weeks achieved similarly high rates of SVR regardless of baseline RAS status. All GT1b with and without pretreatment RASs achieved an SVR after 12 weeks of PrOD (no RBV).

Elbasvir/Grazoprevir

EBR/GZR is another STR recently approved for genotype 1 and 4 chronic HCV infection. It consists of a second-generation PI (GZR) and an NS5A inhibitor (EBR) that has been shown to have high rates of viral cure among many patient types including treatment-naive and -experienced, both with and without cirrhosis, and those with end-stage renal failure.[43–45] Data from the studies described next informed the decision to include pretreatment RAS testing to the prescribing label. Patients with genotype 1a infection (approximately 10%–12% of the genotype 1a population), but not 1b, found to have baseline NS5A RASs should have their treatment extended and combined with RBV to maximize the chance of cure.[46]

In the C-EDGE treatment-naive study,[43] genotype 1 patients with and without cirrhosis were treated for 12 weeks with EBR/GZR. There was no impact on SVR observed among those patients with and without NS3 baseline RASs. NS5A baseline RASs were observed in 12% (19 of 154) of the GT1a patients. Only 58% (11 of 19) of these patients achieved SVR compared with 99% (133 of 135) of those without baseline NS5A RASs. Fourteen percent (18 of 130) of GT1b were found to have baseline NS5A RASs, but no difference in rate of SVR was observed between those with (94%; 17 of 18) and those without (100%; 112 of 112) pretreatment substitutions.[3]

In the C-EDGE treatment-experienced study, genotype 1, 4, and 6 patients who failed prior peginterferon and RBV, with and without cirrhosis, were enrolled. Participants were randomized to one of four arms and treated with EBR/GZR for 12 or 16 weeks with and without RBV. Again, the presence of NS3 RASs did not reduce SVR rates in either GT1a or 1b patients. Patients without baseline NS5A RASs had universally high rates of SVR (>98%) regardless of genotype. In patients with GT1b, the presence or absence of baseline NS5A RASs had no effect on rate of SVR (93.3% [28 of 30] vs 100% [117 of 117]). Although this was also true for individuals with GT4 (n = 37) and GT6 (n = 6), the number of individuals included in the study with these rarer genotypes was low. For GT1a, NS5A pretreatment RASs had a clear impact on SVR; 99% (190 of 192) of those without a baseline substitution compared with 67.7% (21 of 31) of those with a variant achieved cure. The effect of baseline NS5A RASs varied with study treatment arm; in those GT1a patients with baseline NS5A RASs treated with 12 weeks of EVR/GZR alone the rate of SVR was 60%, whereas 100% (six of six) of similar patients were cured with 16 weeks of EZR/GZR with RBV.[45]

A recent pooled assessment of resistance data from phase 2 and 3 EVR/GZR studies was presented[47] and included data from 960 GT1a or 1b treatment-naive and experienced patients with and without cirrhosis, chronic kidney disease, and human immunodeficiency virus coinfection. This analysis affirmed that baseline RASs in the NS3 gene had no impact on treatment outcome. NS5A RASs did not affect the rate of cure in treatment-naive or experienced GT1b patients who relapsed after peginterferon and RBV. For GT1a patients treated with only 12 weeks of EZR/GZR without RBV, a 12% reduction in SVR was observed in those with baseline NS5A RASs (86%; 74 of 86) compared with those without (98%; 345 of 352) these substitutions. The rate of SVR was even further reduced to 58% (14 of 24) when only EZR-specific RASs were considered, particularly those at NS5A positions 30, 31, and 93.

A total of 100% of patients regardless of NS5A or EZR-specific RASs, however, achieved SVR when treated with 16 or 18 weeks of EZR/GZR with RBV.

These findings have led to the recommendation in the US label for EBR/GZR, also reflected in the American Association for the Study of Liver Diseases Guidelines, that patients with genotype 1a be tested for baseline RASs before use of this regimen and, if present at the 28, 30, 31, and/or 93 positions, 16 weeks of EBR/GZR with RBV should be administered.[48]

Sofosbuvir/Velpatasvir

The phase 3 ASTRAL studies demonstrated the efficacy of a simple, once-daily, pan-genotypic STR of coformulated SOF/VEL in a broad range of HCV populations and genotypes.[49] The high potency of this regimen seems to mitigate the impact of baseline RASs, except for patients with genotype 3 infection or those with decompensated cirrhosis.

In ASTRAL-1, a total of 624 patients with genotypes 1a, 1b, 2, 4, 5, or 6 were enrolled with an overall success rate of 99%.[50] There were only two virologic failures, both caused by relapse. Given the high rate of cure, it is not surprising that the presence of pretreatment NS5A RASs did not seem to impact treatment outcome. Although both patients with virologic failure had a pretreatment NS5A RAS, 255 of the 257 (99%) individuals with baseline NS5A substitutions achieved an SVR.[50]

ASTRAL-3 was an independent study restricted to treatment-naive and experienced patients with genotype 3 infection.[51] Overall, 95% of patients treated with 12 weeks of SOF/VEL achieved SVR. There were 11 virologic failures and a signal was raised, however, that baseline RASs may impact the efficacy of SOF/VEL in genotype 3 patients. Only 38 of 43 (88%) of GT3 patients with baseline RASs had an SVR. By contrast, 225 of the 231 (97%) patients without a baseline RAS had an SVR.

The ATRAL 4 study was an open-label study that evaluated the safety and efficacy of SOF/VEL in 287 patients decompensated Childs class B cirrhosis.[52] Given the small study, a complete analysis of the impact that NS5A resistance had on SVR in these patients with decompensated cirrhosis was not performed. Still, it seemed that assessing for NS5A resistance and adding RBV when present may be a reasonable strategy to maximize cure in this complicated HCV population. Rates of SVR 12 in genotype 1 patients with and without pretreatment NS5A RASs were 100% and 98% in those who received SOF/VEL with RBV. In those treated with SOF/VEL alone for 12 or 24 weeks, the rates of SVR were 80% versus 96% and 90% versus 98%, respectively. Because of the small sample size, the impact of NS5A RASs in genotype 3 patients was not established. The advantage that adding RBV has in enhancing rates of cure in decompensated cirrhosis needs further investigation in larger studies.

These findings were summarized and emphasized in a recent analysis of resistance among all patients in the ASTRAL clinical program demonstrating that baseline RASs, particularly the Y93N/H variant, significantly reduced SVR in genotype 3 but had no impact on SVR in patients with genotype 1, 2, 4, 5, or 6 infection.[53] Moreover, although virologic failure was rare (1.1%), 14 of the 15 patients who relapsed had viral populations enriched with the Y93N/H mutation.[53]

RETREATMENT AFTER FAILURE OF DIRECT-ACTING ANTIVIRAL THERAPY

As combinations of DAA become more effective, the number of individuals who fail interferon-free therapy is expected to be small. Small studies have demonstrated that, in principle, these patients can be cured when rechallenged with combinations of DAA with or without RBV.[54] Recently, results from the POLARIS-1 trial were presented in which NS5A inhibitor–experienced patients were treated with a 12-week salvage regimen of SOF/VEL/voxilaprevir.[55] Overall, 96% of patients achieved SVR (253 of 263) including 96% (97 of 101), 100% (45 of 45), and 95% (74 of 78) of individuals with genotype 1a, 1b, and 3 infection. As expected with prior NS5A exposure and failure, a large percentage of individuals had baseline NS5A RASs (79%). However, the presence of these substitutions did not seem to reduce the efficacy of the triple regimen because rates of SVR in those with (94%; 120 of 127) and without NS5A RASs (98%; 42 of 43) were similar. In addition, two patients had the signature S282T high-level SOF resistance substitution before retreatment and both achieved SVR. The role of RASs in retreatment of DAA failures is likely to become even less relevant with more potent DAA combinations. In the treatment-naive POLARIS-2 study,[56] patients who had virologic failure after 8 weeks of SOF/VEL/voxilaprevir did not develop treatment-emergent RASs, in contradistinction to observations in patients who fail a dual NS5A/SOF regimen.

RESISTANCE TESTING IN CLINICAL PRACTICE
Pretreatment Resistance-Associated Substitutions Testing

Pretreatment testing for baseline RASs before initiation of antiviral therapy is an important and powerful tool that could guide treatment selection in certain patient populations. Currently there are several commercial reference laboratories that offer reliable baseline population-based RAS testing. These facilities report variants when present in approximately 15% or more of the quasispecies with turnaround times of just a few days, allowing clinicians to make swift treatment optimization decisions.

Nonetheless, the role of RAS testing in clinical practice is only now emerging and it is premature to advise universal baseline testing before treatment. For genotype 1a patients, however, there are consistent signals of reduced SVR when baseline RASs are present, especially when there is a history of prior treatment failure or cirrhosis. Presently, baseline RAS testing of genotype 1a patients (and intensifying therapy with RBV when identified) is only mandated when considering EZR/GZR. Additional studies are needed to determine if this approach should be generalized to other treatment regimens.

The PrOD regimen obviates baseline testing because, per the label, all genotype 1a patients are treated with RBV for 12 (noncirrhotic) or 24 weeks (compensated cirrhosis) regardless of NS5A status. There is also no recommendation for baseline testing before LDV/SOF treatment, although in some instances clinicians may elect to do so. Given the recent analysis demonstrating reduced SVR in treatment-experienced and cirrhotic genotype 1a patients, there may be a role of testing and potentially extending therapy or adding RBV to these patient subsets when NS5A substitutions are identified.[3]

There are no label-specific recommendations for baseline RAS testing before treatment with SOF/VEL. In genotype 1a the presence of NS5A baseline RASs did not reduce SVR; there were too few virologic failures to assess if prior treatment failure or advanced liver disease patients would benefit from RAS testing. In genotype 3, although not a label-specific recommendation, the American Association for the Study of Liver Diseases Guidelines advise testing for RASs and adding RBV when the Y93 polymorphism is detected in treatment (interferon)-experienced patients without cirrhosis and treatment-naive patients with cirrhosis, and simply adding RBV in treatment-experienced patients with cirrhosis.[48] There are no recommendations for extending treatment duration beyond 12 weeks with SOF/VEL.

Resistance-Associated Substitutions Testing at Time of Treatment Failure and Before Retreatment

At the time of virologic failure, the presence of treatment-emergent RASs in the NS5A class is nearly universal. Resistance testing at the time of relapse of viral breakthrough is not clinically meaningful and therefore resistance testing need not be performed,[2] although many clinicians including the authors do obtain such testing in these patients. There are insufficient data to guide retreatment after DAA failure and salvage therapies are being evaluated. Current guidelines advise waiting for results of clinical studies before retreatment. For patients with an urgent need for retreatment, it is reasonable to perform resistance testing and use these data to assist in the selection of DAA agents and the duration of treatment.

PERSPECTIVE

Interferon-free DAA regimens have vastly transformed the HCV landscape and the promise of cure is within reach for all patients living with chronic HCV infection. Combinations of inhibitors already have the power to cure more than 90% of patients and additional combinations of next-generation DAAs are just around the corner. The role of RAS testing is slowly emerging; these substitutions clearly have a negative impact on the chance of cure in specific HCV populations, particularly genotype 1a and 3 patients with prior treatment failure and advanced liver disease, and in these settings pretreatment RAS testing and modification of treatment is appropriate. Because the effect of these RASs can seemingly be abrogated by extending or intensifying treatment (with either RBV or next-generation DAAs that possess a higher barrier to resistance), it is possible that any degree of HCV resistance could be overcome with longer duration or more potent treatments.

REFERENCES

1. Jacobson IM. The HCV treatment revolution continues: resistance considerations, pangenotypic efficacy, and advanced in challenging populations. Gastroenterol Hepatol 2016;12(Suppl 10):1–11.
2. Pawlotsky JM. Hepatitis C Virus resistance to direct acting antiviral drugs in interferon-free regimens. Gastroenterology 2016;151:70–86.
3. Zeuzem S, Mizokami M, Pianko S, et al. NS5A resistance-associated substitutions in patients with genotype 1 hepatitis C virus: prevalence and effect on treatment outcome. J Hepatol 2017;66(5):910–8.
4. Escheverria N, Moratorio G, Cristina J, et al. Hepatitis C virus genetic variability and evolution. World J Hepatol 2014;7:831–45.
5. Smith DB, Bukh J, Muerhoff AS, et al. Expanded classification of hepatitis C virus into 7 genotypes and 67 subtypes: updated criteria and genotype assignment web resource. Hepatology 2014;59:318–27.
6. Bartenschlager R, Lohmann V. Replication of hepatitis C virus. J Gen Virol 2000; 81:1631–48.
7. Martel M, Esteban JI, Quer J, et al. Hepatitis C virus (HCV) circulated as a population of different but closely related genomes: quasispecies nature of HCV genome distribution. J Virol 1992;66:3225–9.
8. Laskus T, Wilkinson J, Gallegos-Orozco JF. Analysis of hepatitis C virus quasispecies transmission and evolution in patients infected through blood transfusion. Gastroenterology 2004;127:764–76.

9. Sarrazin C, Zeuzem S. Resistance to direct antiviral agents in patients with hepatitis C virus infection. Gastroenterology 2010;138:447–62.

10. Poveda E, Wyles DL, Pedreidra JD, et al. Updated on hepatitis C virus resistance to direct-acting antiviral agents. Antiviral Res 2014;108:181–91.

11. Qi X, Bae A, Liu S, et al. Development of a replicon based phenotypic assay for assessing the drug susceptibilities of HCV NS3 protease genes from clinical isolates. Antiviral Res 2009;81:166–73.

12. Rupp D, Dietz J, Sikorski AM, et al. A phenotypic NS-3 protease inhibitor resistance assays to characterize resistance associated mutations in patients. J Viral Hepat 2015;22:93.

13. Sarrazin C. The importance of resistance to direct antiviral drugs in HCV infection in clinical practice. J Hepatol 2016;64:486–504.

14. Dietz J, Schelhorn SE, Fitting D, et al. Deep sequencing reveals mutagenic effects of ribavirin during monotherapy of hepatitis C virus genotype 1 infected patients. J Virol 2013;87:6172–81.

15. Susser S, Beggel B, Perner D, et al. Comparison of three sequencing methods commonly used in hepatitis C virus resistance analysis: population-based vs. clonal-based vs. ultra deep sequencing. J Hepatol 2015;62:S679.

16. Lontok E, Harrington P, Howe A, et al. Hepatitis C virus drug resistance associated substitutions: state of the art summary. Hepatology 2015;62:1623–32.

17. Romano KP, Ali A, Aydin C, et al. The molecular basis of drug resistance against hepatitis C virus NS3/4A protease inhibitors. PLoS Pathog 2012;8:e1002832.

18. Kuntzen T, Timm J, Berical A, et al. Naturally occurring dominant resistance mutations to hepatitis C virus protease and polymerase inhibitors in treatment naïve patients. Hepatology 2008;48:1769–78.

19. Bartels DJ, Sullivan JC, Zhang EZ, et al. Hepatitis C variants with decreased sensitivity to direct acting antivirals (DAAs) were rarely observed in DAA naive patients prior to treatment. J Virol 2013;87:1544–53.

20. Lenz O, Verbinnen T, Fevery B, et al. Virology analyses of HCV isolates from genotype 1 infected patients treated with simeprevir plus peginterferon/ribavirin in phase IIb/III studies. J Hepatol 2015;62:1008–14.

21. Vincenti I, Rose A, Saladini F, et al. Naturally occurring hepatitis C virus (HCV) NS3/4A protease inhibitor resistance-related mutations in HCV genotype 1 infected subjects in Italy. J Antimicrob Chemother 2012;67:984–7.

22. De Carvahlo IM, Alves R, de Souza PA, et al. Protease inhibitor resistance mutations in untreated Brazilian patients infected with HCV: novel insights about targeted genotyping approaches. J Med Virol 2014;86:1714–21.

23. Sarrazin C, Lathouwers E, Peeters M, et al. Prevalence of the hepatitis C virus NS3 polymorphism Q80K in genotype 1 patients in the European region. Antiviral Res 2015;116:10–6.

24. Sarrazin C, Dvory-Sobol H, Svarocskaia ES, et al. Prevalence of resistance associated substitutions in HCV NS5A, NS5B, or NS3 and outcomes of treatment with ledipasvir and sofosbuvir. Gastroenterology 2016;151:501–12.

25. Zeuzem S, Dusheiko GM, Salupere R, et al. Sofosbuvir and ribavirin in HCV genotype 2 and 3. N Engl J Med 2014;370:1993–2001.

26. Svarovskaia ES, Dvory-Sobol H, Parkin N, et al. Infrequent development of resistance in genotype 1-6 hepatitis C patients treated with sofosbuvir in phase 2 and 3 clinical trials. Clin Infect Dis 2014;59:1666–74.

27. Gane EJ, Abergek AM, Metevier S, et al. The emergence of NS5B resistant associated variant S282T after sofosbuvir based treatment. Hepatology 2015;62:S322A.

28. Hedskog C, Dvory-Sobol H, Gontcharova V, et al. Evolution of the HCV viral population from a patient with S282T detected at relapse after sofosbuvir monotherapy. J Viral Hepat 2015;22:871–81.

29. Svarovskaia ES, Dvory-Sobol H, Doehle B, et al. L159F and V321A sofosbuvir associated hepatitis C virus NS5B substitutions. J Infect Dis 2016;213:1240–7.

30. Krishnan P, Tripathi R, Schnell G, et al. Resistance analysis of baseline and treatment-emergent variants in hepatitis C virus genotype 1 in the AVIATOR study with paritaprevir-ritonavir, ombitasvir, and dasabuvir. Antimocrob Agents Chemother 2015;59:5445–54.

31. Krishnan P, Tripathi R, Schnell G, et al. Long-term follow up of treatment emergent resistance associated variants in NS3, NS5A, and NS5B with paritparevir/ritonavir, ombitasvir, and dasabuvir based regimens. J Hepatol 2015;62:S220.

32. Dvory-Sobol H, Wyles D, Ouyang W, et al. Long term persistence of NCV NS5A variants after treatment with NS5A inhibitor ledipasvir. J Hepatol 2015;62:S221.

33. Afdhal N, Zeuzem S, Kwo P, et al. Ledipasvir and sofosbuvir for untreated genotype 1 infection. N Engl J Med 2014;370:1889–98.

34. Afdhal N, Reddy KR, Nelson DR, et al. Ledipasvir and sofosbuvir for previously treated HCV genotype 1 infection. N Engl J Med 2014;370:1483–93.

35. Kowdley KV, Gordon SC, Reddy KR, et al. Ledipasvir and sofosbuvir for 8 or 12 weeks in chronic HCV without cirrhosis. N Engl J Med 2014;370:1879–88.

36. Lawitz EJ, Poordad FF, Pang PS, et al. Sofosbuvir and ledipasvir fixed dose combination with and without ribavirin in treatment-naive and previously treated patients with genotype 1 hepatitis C virus infection (Lonestar): an open label, randomized phase 2 trial. Lancet 2014;383:515–23.

37. Kowdley KV, Lawitz E, Poordad D, et al. Phase 2b trial of interferon free therapy for hepatitis C virus genotype 1. N Engl J Med 2014;370:222–32.

38. Feld JJ, Kowdley KV, Coakley E, et al. Treatment of HCV with ABT-450/r-ombitasvir and dasabuvir with ribavirin. N Engl J Med 2014;370:1594–603.

39. Zeuzem S, Jacobson IM, Baykal T, et al. Retreatment of HCV with ABT-450/r-ombitasvir and dasabuvir with ribavirin. N Engl J Med 2014;370:1604–14.

40. Ferenci P, Bernstein D, Lalezari J, et al. ABT-450/r-ombitasvir and dasabuvir with or without ribavirin for HCV. N Engl J Med 2014;370:1983–92.

41. Krishnan P, Tripathi R, Schnell G, et al. Pooled analysis of resistance in patients treated with ombitasvir/ABT-450r/and dasabuvir with or without ribavirin in phase 2 and 3 clinical trials. Hepatology 2014;60:1134a–5a.

42. Sulkowski M, Krishnan P, Tripathi R, et al. Effect of baseline resistance associated variants on SVR with the 3D regimen plus RBV. Abstract. Conference on retroviruses and opportunistic infections (CROI). Boston (MA), February 22–25, 2016.

43. Zeuzem S, Ghalib R, Reddy KR, et al. Grazoprevir-elbasvir combination therapy for treatment naive cirrhotic and noncirrhotic patients with chronic hepatitis C virus genotype 1, 4, or 6 infection: a randomized trial. Ann Intern Med 2015;163:1–13.

44. Roth D, Nelson DR, Bruchfeld A, et al. Grazoprevir plus elbasvir in treatment naive and treatment experienced patients with hepatitis C virus genotype 1 infection and stage 4-5 chronic kidney disease (the C-SURFER study): a combination phase 3 study. Lancet 2015;386:1537–45.

45. Kwo PE, Gane E, Peng CY, et al. Efficacy and safety of grazoprevir/elbasvir +/- RBV for 12 weeks in patients with HCV G1 or G4 infection who previously failed peginterferon/RBV: C-EDGE treatment-experienced trial. Gastroenterology 2017; 152:164–75.

46. Zepatier prescribing information. Available at: https://www.merck.com/product/usa/pi_circulars/z/zepatier/zepatier_pi.pdf. Accessed March 15, 2017.
47. Jacobson IM, Asante-Appiah E, Wong P, et al. Prevalence and impact of baseline NS5A resistance associated variants (RAVS) on the efficacy of elbasvir/grazoprevir (EBR/GZR) against genotype 1a infection. Hepatology 2015;62:1393A.
48. AASLD-IDSA. Recommendations for testing, managing, and treating hepatitis C. Available at: http://www.hcvguidelines.org. Accessed March 15, 2017.
49. Asselah T, Charlton M, Feld J, et al. The ASTRAL studies: evaluation of SOF/GS-5816 single-tablet regimen for the treatment of genotype 1-6 HCV infection. Vienna (Austria): European Association for the Study of the Liver (EASL); 2015.
50. Feld JJ, Jacobson IM, Hezode C, et al. Sofosbuvir and velpatasvir for HCV genotype 1, 2, 4, 5, and 6 infection. N Engl J Med 2016;373(27):2599–607.
51. Foster GR, Afdhal N, Roberts SK, et al. Sofosbuvir and velpatasvir for HCV genotype 2 and 3 infection. N Engl J Med 2015;373(27):2608–17.
52. Curry MP, O'Leary JG, Bzowej N, et al. Sofosbuvir and velpatasvir for HCV in patients with decompensated cirrhosis. N Engl J Med 2016;373:2618–28.
53. Hezode C, Chevaliez S, Scoazec G, et al. Retreatment with sofosbuvir and simeprevir of patients with hepatitis C virus genotype 1 or 4 who previously failed daclatasvir containing regimen. Hepatology 2016;63:1809–16.
54. Hezode C, Reau N, Svarovskaia ES, et al. Resistance analysis in 1284 patients with genotype 1-6 HCV infection treated with sofosbuvir/velpatasvir in the phase 3 ASTRAL-1, ASTRAL-2, ASTRAL-3, and ASTRAL-4 studies. Barcelona (Spain): European Association for the Study of the Liver (EASL); 2016.
55. Bourliere M, Gordon S, Alnoor R, et al. Sofosbuvir/velpastasvir/voxilaprevir for 12 weeks as a salvage regimen in NS5A inhibitor-experienced patients with genotypes 1-6 infection; the phase 3 POLARIS-1 study. Boston: AASLD; 2016.
56. Jacobson IM, Asselah T, Nahass R, et al. A randomized phase 3 trial of sofosbuvir/velpatasvir/voxilaprevir for 8 weeks compared to sofosbuvir/velpatasvir for 12 weeks in DAA-naive genotype 1-6 HCV infected patients: the POLARIS-2 study. Boston: AASLD; 2016.

Genetic Testing in Liver Disease
What to Order, in Whom, and When

Emily A. Schonfeld, MD, Robert S. Brown Jr, MD, MPH*

KEYWORDS

- Genetic testing • Hemochromatosis • Wilson disease
- Progressive familial intrahepatic cholestasis
- Benign recurrent intrahepatic cholestasis • Lysosomal acid lipase deficiency
- Gilbert syndrome • Alpha-1 antitrypsin deficiency

KEY POINTS

- The most common cause of hereditary hemochromatosis is a C282Y mutation in the HFE gene with a penetrance of 10% to 52%.
- Gilbert syndrome is a common and benign cause of indirect hyperbilirubinemia with no signs of hemolysis and no associated liver injury.
- Progressive familial intrahepatic cholestasis is a rare cause of chronic cholestasis in children and young adults. Benign recurrent intrahepatic cholestasis is a benign cause of recurrent cholestasis seen in both adults and children.
- Alpha-1 antitrypsin deficiency causes both lung and liver disease. It is the most common genetic cause of liver disease in children.
- Wilson disease can cause neurologic disease and liver disease. Patients between the ages of 3 and 55 years with any acute or unexplained chronic liver disease should be tested for Wilson disease.

INTRODUCTION

When evaluating a patient with abnormal liver function tests, investigating genetic causes of liver disease is an important part of the work-up. The initial evaluation of a patient with abnormal liver function tests includes a history and physical examination. Family history plays a critical role because it can help determine which patients to consider for genetic testing. The age of onset of abnormal liver function tests and the pattern of abnormal liver function tests, hepatocellular or cholestatic, play a role

Disclosures: The authors have nothing to disclose.
Transitions of Care, Division of Gastroenterology and Hepatology, Weill Cornell Medical College, Center for Liver Disease, 1305 York Avenue, 4th Floor, New York, NY 10021, USA
* Corresponding author.
E-mail address: rsb2005@med.cornell.edu

in what testing is performed. This article evaluates common genetic causes of liver disease, when and in whom to test for them, and what tests to order.

HEREDITARY HEMOCHROMATOSIS

Hemochromatosis occurs from the unregulated transfer of iron from the intestine into the blood leading to toxic levels depositing in various organs and is usually caused by an underlying genetic disorder.[1] Most (80%–90%) cases of hereditary hemochromatosis are caused by an autosomal recessive mutation in the *HFE* gene, C282Y.[2–8] Two less common mutations are H63D and S65C, which usually only cause signs and symptoms of iron overload when present as compound heterozygotes with C282Y.[2,4,9] In patients with liver disease, 3% to 5.3% are homozygous for C282Y and therefore testing for hemochromatosis should be performed in the work-up of liver disease of unknown cause or in patients with iron overload on laboratory testing or imaging.[5,9] It is especially important to test those patients who have a first-degree relative with hereditary hemochromatosis as well as those patients with imaging studies that show iron overload.[2,5,8] At diagnosis, about 4.4% to 11.8% of C282Y homozygous male patients have cirrhosis and 0% to 2.7% of C282Y female patients have cirrhosis.[1,7,10] Therefore early diagnosis is important because initiation of phlebotomy before the development of cirrhosis can reduce or stop the progression of hereditary hemochromatosis.[2,10]

Hereditary hemochromatosis is most commonly seen in Caucasian of Northern European descent.[2,6,9] About 6% to 10% of Caucasian have 1 allele for C282Y and 1 in 250 to 300 Caucasian have 2 alleles.[1,4,5] Although the HFE gene mutations are fairly common, only 10% to 52% of patients homozygous for C282Y develop clinical signs of iron overload.[1,2,5–8,11] Manifestations of hereditary hemochromatosis are more prevalent in men and present earlier in men, likely in part because of menstruation and therefore iron loss in women.[2,5,6,8,10] Patients with hereditary hemochromatosis can show other symptoms of iron overload that may prompt testing, such as chondrocalcinosis, diabetes mellitus type 1, heart failure, or porphyria cutanea tarda[1,2,5,6] Up to 19% of patients with porphyria cutanea tarda are homozygous for C282Y.[5,8,12]

The initial screening tests for hereditary hemochromatosis include blood tests for ferritin and transferrin saturation, which is calculated from iron/total iron binding capacity.[2,5] Transferrin saturation greater than 45% should prompt genetic testing for the most common causes of hereditary hemochromatosis.[1,2,4–6,9] An increased ferritin level is also expected in hereditary hemochromatosis, but is not highly specific, thus an increased ferritin level with a normal transferrin saturation is not common in hereditary hemochromatosis and should lead to investigation into alternative causes of liver disease.[1,13] In hereditary hemochromatosis, a ferritin level is still useful because of its high sensitivity and because a level greater than 1000 μg/L can help predict patients who have advanced fibrosis.[2,10] Testing for advanced fibrosis or cirrhosis should be performed in patients who are homozygous for C282Y or compound heterozygotes for C282Y who have a ferritin greater than 1000 μg/L, hepatomegaly, age more than 40 years, or abnormal liver tests.[2,5,6,10,14] A liver biopsy is not always necessary because MRI can evaluate for cirrhotic morphology and can quantify the amount of iron in the liver, and transient elastography can also be used to evaluate for advanced fibrosis.[5,15,16]

In patients with laboratory testing consistent with iron overload, but who are not C282Y homozygotes, other causes of liver disease should be considered.[1,2,15] Iron overload is common in other liver diseases, such as alcohol-related liver disease, nonalcoholic fatty liver disease (NAFLD) and viral hepatidites.[1,2,13,15,17] In this situation, a liver biopsy may be necessary to investigate for alternative causes of liver disease.[2] In these patients, heterozygosity or compound heterozygosity for C282Y or H63D may lead to more advanced liver disease because of increased iron stores.[3] Liver biopsies should be stained with Perls Prussian blue to determine the amount of iron and the location of iron present.[2,15] Iron overload can be seen in cirrhosis of any cause; however, in hemochromatosis, the distinguishing feature is that iron is deposited in the fibrous septa, bile ducts, and walls of the vasculature.[15] The hepatic iron concentration in a liver biopsy of at least 236 μmol/g dry weight has a sensitivity of 80% and a specificity of 78% for distinguishing patients with cirrhosis.[2,10]

If true hepatic iron overload is present, non-HFE genetic hemochromatosis should be suspected. Less common genetic causes of hereditary hemochromatosis include juvenile hemochromatosis, mutations in transferrin receptor-2, mutations in ferroportin, aceruloplasminemia, atransferrinemia, and African iron overload.[2,18] Given the rarity of these mutations, genetic testing for the disorders is infrequently performed.[1,5,15] Genetic testing is only done if laboratory analysis suggests iron overload, but *HFE* mutations and other causes of liver disease are ruled out or treated and iron overload in the liver is confirmed.[1,5,15] In contrast with *HFE*-associated hereditary hemochromatosis, ferroportin disease and aceruloplasminemia show a transferrin saturation less than 45% with an increased ferritin level and signs of iron overload.[5] These findings need to be distinguished from secondary iron overload caused by excessive dietary intake or hemolysis/ineffective erythropoiesis.

Disease	Common Laboratory Abnormalities	Presentation of Disease
Hereditary hemochromatosis (*HFE* form)	↑AST/ALT Transferrin saturation >45% ↑Ferritin Genotype analysis most commonly C282Y homozygote	Abnormal LFTs Cirrhosis Type 1 diabetes mellitus Heart failure
What test to order? *HFE* genotype		

Abbreviations: ALT, alanine transaminase; AST, aspartate transaminase; LFTs, liver function tests.

GILBERT SYNDROME

Gilbert syndrome is a benign cause of unconjugated hyperbilirubinemia in people with no liver disease or hemolysis.[19] It is caused by reduced bilirubin glucuronidation, a process needed to excrete bilirubin. The prevalence is about 1.6% to 10% of the population.[19–21] The bilirubin levels can fluctuate, but are usually between 1 and 5 mg/dL, always with a normal direct (conjugated) bilirubin level.[19,20,22,23] In adults, it does not lead to clinically significant liver disease.[19,21] Patients have normal aminotransferase and alkaline phosphatase levels, and their hemolysis work-up is negative with no other physical examination findings to suggest liver disease.[19,22] In studies that have evaluated liver biopsies in these patients, normal histology was noted, and a liver biopsy is not needed for diagnosis.[22] Thus patients with isolated unconjugated hyperbilirubinemia and no other evidence of liver disease should be reassured and require no further work-up. Gilbert syndrome is more prevalent in men than in women and fasting can increase the serum bilirubin level.[19,21]

Disease	Common Laboratory Abnormalities	Presentation of Disease
Gilbert syndrome	+Unconjugated bilirubin	Fasting increases bilirubin level

PROGRESSIVE FAMILIAL INTRAHEPATIC CHOLESTASIS

Progressive familial intrahepatic cholestasis (PFIC) encompasses 3 autosomal recessive mutations that lead to chronic cholestasis: PFIC1, PFIC2, and PFIC3.[24] The incidence of PFIC is about 1 per 50,000 to 1 per 100,000 births, and it is the cause of liver disease in about 10% to 15% of children with cholestatic liver tests.[24–28] Patients with PFIC can present with jaundice, pruritus, splenomegaly, and hepatomegaly.[24,25,29] Specifically, patients with PFIC1 and PFIC2 usually present at a few months of age, whereas patients with PFIC3 usually present later in childhood or early adulthood.[24,25,29] Despite cholestatic abnormalities on their liver tests, patients with PFIC1 and PFIC2 have normal gamma-glutamyltransferase (GGT) levels, whereas patients with PFIC3 have increased GGT levels.[24,25,29] All 3 classifications of PFIC have increased serum bile acid levels.[24,25,29]

PFIC1 and PFIC3 usually present with a mild increase in alanine transaminase (ALT) level and a normal alpha fetoprotein (AFP) level, whereas patients with PFIC2 show a marked increase in ALT level to more than 5 times normal with an increased AFP level.[24,30] PFIC1 and PFIC2 often present at a few months of age with recurrent or chronic jaundice and PFIC2 usually progresses more quickly than PFIC1 to end-stage liver disease.[24,30] Hepatocellular carcinoma or cholangiocarcinoma at a very young age (<1 year old) can be seen in PFIC2 and therefore, after diagnosis, screening for malignancies with imaging modalities is important.[24–26,30] Patients with PFIC1 can have other signs of the disease, such as short height, deafness, diarrhea, pancreatitis, an increased sweat electrolyte concentration, and hepatic steatosis.[24,30] In PFIC1, a mutation in the gene ATP8B1, which encodes for the protein FIC1, not only affects the protein expression in the liver but also in the pancreas and small intestine, likely leading to the other symptoms associated with the disease.[29,31] PFIC3 usually presents with cirrhosis later in childhood or young adulthood.[24]

PFIC should be considered in children with cholestasis after more common liver diseases and biliary diseases have been excluded, such as biliary atresia, Alagille syndrome, alpha-1 antitrypsin deficiency, cystic fibrosis, sclerosing cholangitis, and biliary obstruction.[24,25,29] Serum bile acid level should be tested because increased serum bile acid levels rule out problems with bile acid synthesis.[24–26,30] Liver function tests, GGT, and imaging studies help to rule out other more common causes of liver disease before diagnosing PFIC.[24,25,27]

A liver biopsy may aid in the diagnosis of PFIC. A liver biopsy in PFIC1 and PFIC2 commonly shows canalicular cholestasis.[24,25] A liver biopsy in PFIC2 usually shows more fibrosis than is seen in PFIC1 and a giant cell hepatitis.[24,25] A liver biopsy in PFIC3 usually shows proliferation of the bile ducts and fibrosis.[24] Specialized stains can further help differentiate PFIC2 and PFIC3. The gene ABCB11 encodes the bile salt export pump (BSEP) protein, most commonly thought to be defective in PFIC2.[29] The gene ABCB4 encodes the multidrug resistance 3 (MDR3) protein, most commonly thought to be defective in PFIC3.[29] A liver biopsy can be stained for BSEP and MDR3 and therefore differentiate which type of PFIC is present.[24,25,29,30] The protein staining is expected to be low or absent in most PFIC cases; however, normal protein staining may be present if patients have a loss of function mutation with normal synthesis of the proteins, and loss of staining can be infrequently seen in other causes of neonatal cholestasis.[24,25,29,30] Additional testing that may aid in the diagnosis of PFIC is evaluation of the composition of bile. This evaluation is usually done if cholangiography is being performed to rule out other causes of disease. A low bile salt concentration is seen in PFIC1 and PFIC2 (lower in PFIC2) and a low phospholipid level is seen in the bile in PFIC3.[24,30] The proteins mutated in PFIC1 and PFIC2 play a role in the secretion of bile, whereas the protein mutated in PFIC3 plays a role in the translocation of phospholipids into bile.[24,30]

Genetic testing can confirm the diagnosis of PFIC, although in a small number of patients the genetic defect may not be elucidated because some genes likely remain unidentified.[24,26,32] Family history is important in the evaluation of PFIC because cases of heterozygous mutations for the PFIC proteins have been found in women who developed intrahepatic cholestasis of pregnancy.[24]

Disease	Common Laboratory Abnormalities	Presentation of Disease
PFIC	+Alkaline phosphatase	Jaundice
	PFIC1: normal GGT	Pruritus
	Low bile salt concentration in bile	Splenomegaly
	PFIC2: normal GGT	Hepatomegaly
	Low bile salt concentration in bile	PFIC1: short height, deafness, diarrhea,
	+ALT	pancreatitis, increased sweat electrolyte
	+AFP	concentration, hepatic steatosis
	PFIC3: +GGT	PFIC2: HCC or cholangiocarcinoma
	Low phospholipid concentration in bile	PFIC3: cirrhosis in late childhood and young adulthood
What test to order? PFIC genotype (ATP8B1, ABCB11, ABCB4 mutations)		

Abbreviations: HCC, hepatocellular carcinoma.

BENIGN RECURRENT INTRAHEPATIC CHOLESTASIS

Benign recurrent intrahepatic cholestasis (BRIC) is an autosomal recessive disease caused by a mutation in the same genes as in PFIC; however, BRIC is a benign disease.[24] BRIC is a rare disease that can present in both childhood and adulthood and leads to recurrent episodes of cholestasis.[33] Each episode of cholestasis can last for a variable amount of time and the time between episodes can range from weeks to years.[31,34] Between episodes, the patients are asymptomatic with normal liver tests.[31,34] During the recurrent episodes of cholestasis, patients with BRIC develop jaundice, pruritus, increased serum bile acid levels, increased alkaline phosphatase levels, a conjugated hyperbilirubinemia, and a low GGT level.[31,33] BRIC, unlike PFIC, does not progress to chronic cholestasis or cirrhosis.[33]

Some patients experience symptoms before the onset of an episode of cholestasis, such as fatigue, nausea, decreased appetite, and pruritus.[31] If a liver biopsy is performed during an episode of cholestasis, it shows cholestasis but no signs of chronic liver disease.[24,31,33] In order to diagnose BRIC, the patient must have at least 2 episodes of cholestasis with a symptom-free interval and alternative causes of cholestasis must be excluded, which usually includes imaging, laboratory tests, and likely a liver biopsy.[31] Case series have shown that some patients note respiratory tract infections before the episodes of cholestasis.[31,34] The diagnosis can be supported by genetic testing, which would show a mutation in the same genes as are mutated in PFIC.[24,31]

Disease	Common Laboratory Abnormalities	Presentation of Disease
BRIC	During episodes of cholestasis: +alkaline phosphatase +Conjugated hyperbilirubinemia +Serum bile acids Normal GGT Between episodes of cholestasis: Liver tests normal	During episode of cholestasis: jaundice Pruritus

LYSOSOMAL ACID LIPASE DEFICIENCY

Lysosomal acid lipase deficiency (LAL-D) is a rare autosomal recessive disorder that leads to problems with cholesterol metabolism.[35] It is a lysosomal storage disorder caused by a lack of, or deficiency in, liposomal acid lipase,[30,31] which ultimately leads to accumulation of cholesterol in different organs and macrophages.[35,36]

LAL-D has different variations. The most severe form of LAL-D is called Wolman disease, which presents in early childhood, usually at 2 to 4 months of age, with symptoms of malabsorption, calcification of the adrenal glands, and hepatomegaly.[35-38] The symptoms of Wolman disease are caused by the location of lipid accumulation, such as in the liver, spleen, adrenal glands, bone marrow, lymph nodes, macrophages, and small intestinal villi.[35,36] Wolman disease has a high mortality in the first year of life.[36,38] Cholesteryl ester storage disease (CESD) is a different form of LAL-D that can present later in childhood or in adulthood and cause hepatosplenomegaly, dyslipidemia, accelerated atherosclerosis, and liver disease.[35,36] Adrenal calcifications can sometimes be seen in this form of the disease.[36] The different LAL-D phenotypes are based on the level of activity of lysosomal acid lipase.[36] Patients with Wolman disease have either no functioning enzyme or less than 1% activity, which is in contrast with CESD, which has a higher level of activity and therefore later onset.[36]

CESD is most common in Caucasian of European descent.[35,36] About half of all cases of CESD are caused by a mutation in the E8SJM gene.[20] Therefore, screening for this genotype showed an estimated prevalence of the disease to be 25 per million in the German population.[20] In North America, the prevalence of CESD is about 0.8 per 100,000 in white and Hispanic populations.[39]

Patients with LAL-D may present with abnormal liver function tests, splenomegaly, and hepatomegaly.[35,36] When evaluating cholesterol levels, these patients have high triglyceride and total cholesterol levels with low high-density lipoprotein (HDL) levels.[35,36,40] Imaging studies can help rule out other causes of liver disease and evaluate for hepatomegaly; splenomegaly; and, in Wolman disease, adrenal gland calcifications.[35,36] After being ruled out for other more common causes of liver disease, a liver biopsy in these patients can show microvesicular steatosis and birefringent cholesterol ester crystals or their remnant crystals in hepatocytes as well as lipids in the Kupffer cells.[4,35,36,38,41,42] Immunostaining can be performed on the liver biopsy specimen for lysosomal proteins and this confirms that the location of lipid deposition is the lysosomes and aids in the diagnosis.[36] The liver biopsy can be mistaken for NAFLD or cryptogenic cirrhosis, which can make it harder to diagnose adults with the disease.[35,36] A dried blood spot is used to determine the peripheral leukocyte LAL activity because a low activity would support the diagnosis of LAL-D.[4,35,36,38,41,42] Genotype analysis is not necessary for diagnosis, but a mutation in LIPA, the gene for LAL, is diagnostic.[35,36,40]

Disease	Common Laboratory Abnormalities	Presentation of Disease
LAL-D	+AST/ALT +Alkaline phosphatase Decreased peripheral leukocyte LAL activity in blood CESD: +Triglycerides +Total cholesterol Low HDL level	Hepatomegaly Splenomegaly Wolman disease: Calcification of the adrenal glands Symptoms of malabsorption
What test to order? *LIPA* genotype		

ALPHA-1 ANTITRYPSIN DEFICIENCY

Alpha-1 antitrypsin is a protease inhibitor (Pi) produced in the liver that works to inhibit neutrophil elastase, which can degrade proteins, especially in the lungs.[43–46] Alpha-1 antitrypsin deficiency is an autosomal recessive mutation that can lead to early-onset panacinar emphysema in smokers (aged 40–60 years) as well as liver disease.[43,45,46] Other rarer manifestations of alpha-1 antitrypsin deficiency include panniculitis, often at sites of trauma, and vasculitis, which is usually c-ANCA (cytoplasmic antineutrophil cytoplasmic antibody) positive.[46–48]

There are multiple variants of the alpha-1 antitrypsin genotype and some of these variants produce normal levels of alpha-1 antitrypsin, whereas some lead to reduced levels.[45] The reduced levels are associated with disease.[45] The null genotype leads to no production of alpha-1 antitrypsin.[45] The normal alpha-1 antitrypsin genotype is labeled MM and severe deficiency is ZZ.[43,49,50] The ZZ genotype most commonly leads to liver disease and accounts for about 0.1% of patients with abnormal alpha-1 antitrypsin genotypes.[43,49,50] Less commonly, the SZ genotype and the M_{malton} genotype can lead to liver disease.[45,51] The prevalence of alpha-1 antitrypsin deficiency is about 1 per 5000 to 1 per 1640 in Caucasian, and heterozygosis for the MZ phenotype occurs in about 2% to 3% of the white population.[43,44,46,49,52]

The genetic defect associated with alpha-1 antitrypsin deficiency changes the enzyme shape so that it is retained in hepatocytes and can be seen on a liver biopsy when stained with periodic acid–Schiff (PAS) stain.[43,44,53] The enzyme appears as PAS-positive, diastase-resistant globules in hepatocytes.[43,44,53]

Patients with alpha-1 antitrypsin deficiency can present with jaundice, hepatitis, hepatomegaly, and/or cirrhosis in children and with abnormal liver tests or cirrhosis in adults.[43–45,52,54] Patients can have increased bilirubin levels and serum aminotransferase levels.[45,52] In children, the liver function tests may normalize at a few months of age, but they should be followed for progression to cirrhosis.[45,52] Adults diagnosed with alpha-1 antitrypsin deficiency often do not show abnormal liver tests or liver disease in childhood.[45] Alpha-1 antitrypsin deficiency is a more common cause of liver disease in men than in women.[51,52,54]

Although alpha-1 antitrypsin deficiency is the most common genetic cause of liver disease in children, most people with this deficiency do not develop liver disease.[43,44,46,51,52] Only about 7% to 20% of children with alpha-1 antitrypsin deficiency PiZZ genotype develop liver disease.[43,44,46,52] Patients with abnormal liver function tests should be evaluated for alpha-1 antitrypsin deficiency, especially if they have a family history of liver disease or emphysema in a nonsmoker. The screening examination evaluates the level of alpha-1 antitrypsin in the blood.[43,46,49] When low levels are found or pretest suspicion is high, further testing for abnormal phenotypes or genotypes is performed.[43,46,49] The PiS and PiZ genotypes can be diagnosed via isoelectric focusing but, if patients do not have these genotypes and still have a low alpha-1 antitrypsin level, evaluating the alpha-1 antitrypsin gene (SERPINA1) for mutations is necessary.[43,46,49] For example, the null genotype cannot be discovered by isoelectric focusing because no protein is made.[43,46,49] Alpha-1 antitrypsin is an acute phase reactant and levels can be increased in the presence of high estrogen levels, which can cause a false-negative test.[43,46,53] Low alpha-1 antitrypsin levels can also be seen in diseases associated with protein loss, such as via the kidneys or gastrointestinal tract.[43] A liver biopsy may be necessary to rule out other causes of liver disease.

All people with a first-degree relative with alpha-1 antitrypsin deficiency should be tested for the deficiency.[43] Heterozygosity for alpha-1 antitrypsin deficiency in the setting of a second cause of liver disease may aid in the progression to cirrhosis.[51] However, there is no therapy for the liver disease associated with alpha-1 antitrypsin deficiency other than transplant, and transplant cures the deficiency.[45,55]

Disease	Common Laboratory Abnormalities	Presentation of Disease
Alpha-1 antitrypsin deficiency	+AST/ALT +Alkaline phosphatase Genotype analysis most commonly ZZ	Early emphysema in smokers Jaundice or hepatitis in children Cirrhosis in children or adults
What test to order? Alpha-1 antitrypsin phenotype/genotype		

WILSON DISEASE

Wilson disease is caused by an autosomal recessive mutation in ATP7B, which helps transport copper into bile and bind copper to ceruloplasmin.[18,56–59] The incidence is as high as 1 per 30,000 and specifically the incidence in an Irish population was estimated at 17 per 1 million births with a prevalence of 3.6 per 1 million people.[18,58–61] The mutation in ATP7B leads to copper deposition in the liver as well as the brain, kidneys, and cornea leading to varying manifestations of the disease.[18,58]

Wilson disease most commonly presents between 5 years old and 40 years old, but it should be considered in patients with liver abnormalities between the ages of 3 and 55 years, especially if a patient has symptoms suggestive of Wilson disease.[58] Patients with Wilson disease can present with no symptoms and a mild increase in aminotransferase levels, hepatomegaly, neurologic symptoms, or acute liver failure with a Coombs-negative hemolytic anemia and acute kidney injury.[58,61–63] Many patients already have cirrhosis at presentation, which is usually present by the second decade of life.[57,58,62,63] A small percentage of patients present with hemolysis alone.[58,61] Similar to autoimmune hepatitis, patients with Wilson disease can have increased immunoglobulin and autoantibody levels.[58] A special population in which Wilson disease should be considered are patients with the diagnosis of autoimmune hepatitis who do not respond quickly to steroid treatment and any pediatric patient with the diagnosis of autoimmune hepatitis.[58,62]

Neurologic changes seen in Wilson disease usually present in the third decade of life, but small changes in childhood, such as handwriting or behavior, can be seen.[57,58,60] The neurologic findings in Wilson disease are usually parkinsonian characteristics, such as rigidity and dystonia, as well as dysarthria, and brain imaging can detect abnormalities in the basal ganglia, although this is not diagnostic.[58,60] Features on MRI brain most consistent with Wilson disease include signal changes in the midbrain tectal plate; changes similar to those seen in central pontine myelinolysis; involvement of the basal ganglia, thalamus, and brainstem at the same time; as well as an image called the face of the giant panda.[64] Patients may also present with psychiatric disorders.[58,60] Patients with neurologic symptoms from Wilson disease usually first have liver disease and are often cirrhotic at the time of diagnosis.[60,65] Any patients with liver disease and neurologic or psychiatric findings should be tested for Wilson disease.[58]

Ceruloplasmin can be used as an initial screening examination for Wilson disease.[66] Ceruloplasmin level less than 20 mg/dL has a sensitivity of 95% and specificity of 84.5% for Wilson disease in children with increased aminotransferase levels.[66] Kayser-Fleischer rings, caused by copper deposition in the cornea and diagnosed by slit-lamp eye examinations, are seen in 44% to 62% of patients with hepatic Wilson disease and in about 85.5% to 95% of patients with neurologic Wilson disease.[57,58,60,67] If low ceruloplasmin level (<20 mg/dL), high 24-hour urine copper level (>40 μg), and Kayser-Fleischer rings are present, then the diagnosis of Wilson disease is confirmed.[57,58,65,66,68] If only 2 of the 3 tests are positive, then a liver biopsy for histology and quantification of copper level (>250 μg/g dry weight of liver) is necessary.[57,58,61] Genetic testing can be performed if patients have an intermediate copper quantification (50–250 μg/g) or if they have an increased urine copper level, Kayser-Fleischer rings, but do not meet the cutoff for copper quantification in the liver.[58]

Wilson disease can be difficult to diagnose. Kayser-Fleischer rings are not specific for Wilson disease because they can be seen in patients with chronic cholestasis from other forms of liver disease.[60,67] The copper quantification cutoff value of 250 μg/g dry weight of liver has a sensitivity 83.3% and a specificity of 98.6% for the diagnosis of Wilson disease.[69] When 75 μg/g dry weight of liver is used as a cutoff, the sensitivity is 96.5% with a decreased specificity of 95.4%.[69] Therefore a level of hepatic copper concentration between 50 and 250 μg/g dry weight of liver should lead to further investigation into the cause of liver disease and it does not rule out Wilson disease.[69] However, copper staining alone is not useful because it is variable in patients with Wilson disease and increased copper binding protein levels can also be seen in cholestasis from other causes.[60,69] Ceruloplasmin is also not a perfect test because it is an acute phase reactant and its levels can be increased in patients with high estrogen levels; for example, during pregnancy.[58,60–62,66,67] Ceruloplasmin level can also be low in patients who are losing proteins via the kidneys or intestines, with lack of production in end-stage liver disease, or with aceruloplasminemia.[58,60,61] Therefore, if ceruloplasmin level is increased but there is still a high suspicion for Wilson disease, a 24-hour urine copper test can aid in diagnosis.[60,66]

In patients who present with acute liver failure caused by Wilson disease, classic findings include Coombs-negative hemolytic anemia, rapidly progressive acute kidney injury, increased serum aminotransferase levels less than 2000 IU/L, and a normal or low alkaline phosphatase test.[58,60–62] Patients who present with acute liver failure usually already have cirrhosis at presentation.[60] The diagnosis of acute Wilson disease is critical because it does not respond to chelation or any medical therapy and thus urgent liver transplant is indicated and the only effective therapy.

A liver biopsy done in patients with Wilson disease can appear similar to biopsies from patients with NAFLD and can show signs of cholestasis, which does not distinguish it from other types of liver disease.[57,58,60,70] The liver biopsy can have iron overload caused by low ceruloplasmin level, which is important in the oxidation and transport of iron, hemolysis, inflammation, and cirrhosis.[15,70] A liver biopsy can help rule out other causes of liver disease.[60] In addition, an increased free serum copper level (not bound to ceruloplasmin) may aid in the diagnosis, although it can be increased in other causes of acute liver failure, cholestatic liver disease, and in a copper overdose.[57,60–62]

Those patients with a first-degree relative with Wilson disease should be tested for the disease.[57,58] Genetic testing can be used as the primary means of diagnosis if the affected relative's genotype is known, because there are multiple mutations on ATP7B that have been identified and patients can be compound heterozygotes.[57,58,60,61] Genotype testing can help confirm the diagnosis in patients with other laboratory tests suggestive of Wilson disease, especially in populations in which certain mutations are more common.[60,65]

Disease	Common Laboratory Abnormalities	Presentation of Disease
Wilson disease	+AST/ALT Low or normal alkaline phosphatase level Low ceruloplasmin level +24-h urine copper +Serum free copper +Hemolysis work-up Genetic analysis with ATP7B mutation	Hepatomegaly Cirrhosis Neurologic symptoms Acute liver failure Kayser-Fleischer rings
What test to order? *ATP7B* genotype		

SUMMARY

Genetic causes of liver disease lead to a wide range of presentations, from mildly abnormal liver tests to acute liver failure. The most common cause of hereditary hemochromatosis is a mutation in the C282Y gene. If this genotype is absent, it is important to rule out other causes of liver disease because alcohol-related liver disease, NAFLD, viral hepatitis, and all causes of cirrhosis can present with blood tests consistent with iron overload.

Gilbert syndrome is a benign cause of indirect hyperbilirubinemia with no signs of hemolysis. PFIC can cause chronic cholestasis and patients usually present between the neonatal period and young adulthood. It is a rare disorder and other causes of cholestasis should be excluded first. Patients with PFIC1 and PFIC2 present with a normal GGT level despite cholestatic liver tests. BRIC is a benign cause of recurrent cholestasis that does not lead to chronic liver disease. Patients with BRIC have a normal GGT level during the episodes of cholestasis.

Patients with Wolman disease, the most severe form of LAL-D, present in childhood and adrenal calcifications are often seen on imaging. Liver biopsies in Wolman disease and CESD show microvesicular steatosis and cholesterol accumulation. The mutation that commonly causes liver disease in alpha-1 antitrypsin deficiency is PiZZ. Patients can present with increased aminotransferase levels, jaundice, and/or cirrhosis. Wilson disease can cause both neurologic disease and liver disease. Patients can present with a spectrum of liver disease from increased aminotransferase levels to fulminant liver failure. In children with abnormal liver tests and positive autoimmune hepatitis serologies, Wilson disease should be ruled out.

REFERENCES

1. Pietrangelo A. Genetics, genetic testing, and management of hemochromatosis: 15 years since hepcidin. Gastroenterology 2015;149(5):1240–51.

2. Bacon BR, Adams PC, Kowdley KV, et al. Diagnosis and management of hemochromatosis: 2011 practice guideline by the American Association for the Study of Liver Diseases. Hepatology 2011;54(1):328–43.

3. Cheng R, Barton JC, Morrison ED, et al. Differences in hepatic phenotype between hemochromatosis patients with *HFE* C282Y homozygosity and other *HFE* genotypes. J Clin Gastroenterol 2009;43(6):569–73.

4. Adams PC, Reboussin DM, Barton JC, et al. Hemochromatosis and iron-overload screening in a racially diverse population. N Engl J Med 2005;352(17):1769–78.

5. European Association For The Study Of The Liver. EASL clinical practice guidelines for HFE hemochromatosis. J Hepatol 2010;53(1):3–22.

6. Allen KJ, Gurrin LC, Constantine CC, et al. Iron-overload-related disease in *HFE* hereditary hemochromatosis. N Engl J Med 2008;358(3):221–30.

7. Gleeson F, Ryan E, Barrett S, et al. Clinical expression of haemochromatosis in Irish C282Y homozygotes identified through family screening. Eur J Gastroenterol Hepatol 2004;16(9):859–63.

8. Bulaj ZJ, Ajioka RS, Phillips JD, et al. Disease-related conditions in relatives of patients with hemochromatosis. N Engl J Med 2000;343(21):1529–35.

9. Poullis A, Moodie SJ, Ang L, et al. Routine transferrin saturation measurement in liver clinic patients increases detection of hereditary haemochromatosis. Ann Clin Biochem 2003;40(Pt 5):521–7.

10. Powell LW, Dixon JL, Ramm GA, et al. Screening for hemochromatosis in asymptomatic subjects with or without a family history. Arch Intern Med 2006;166(3):294–301.

11. Beutler E, Felitti VJ, Koziol JA, et al. Penetrance of 845G–>A (C282Y) HFE hereditary haemochromatosis mutation in the USA. Lancet 2002;359(9302):211–8.

12. Bonkovsky HL, Poh-Fitzpatrick M, Pimstone N, et al. Porphyria cutanea tarda, hepatitis C, and HFE gene mutations in North America. Hepatology 1998;27(6):1661–9.

13. Gordeuk VR, Reboussin DM, McLaren CE, et al. Serum ferritin concentrations and body iron stores in a multicenter, multiethnic primary-care population. Am J Hematol 2008;83(8):618–26.

14. Morrison ED, Brandhagen DJ, Phatak PD, et al. Serum ferritin level predicts advanced hepatic fibrosis among U.S. patients with phenotypic hemochromatosis. Ann Intern Med 2003;138(8):627–33.

15. Deugnier Y, Turlin B. Pathology of hepatic iron overload. Semin Liver Dis 2011;31(3):260–71.

16. Banerjee R, Pavlides M, Tunnicliffe EM, et al. Multiparametric magnetic resonance for the non-invasive diagnosis of liver disease. J Hepatol 2014;60(1):69–77.

17. Nelson JE, Wilson L, Brunt EM, et al. Relationship between pattern of hepatic iron deposition and histologic severity in nonalcoholic fatty liver disease. Hepatology 2011;53(2):448–57.

18. Lv T, Li X, Zhang W, et al. Recent advance in the molecular genetics of Wilson disease and hereditary hemochromatosis. Eur J Med Genet 2016;59(10):532–9.

19. Bosma PJ, Chowdhury JR, Bakker C, et al. The genetic basis of the reduced expression of bilirubin UDP-glucuronosyltransferase I in Gilbert's syndrome. N Engl J Med 1995;333(18):1171–5.

20. Maruo Y, Nakahara S, Yanagi T. Genotype of *UGT1A1* and phenotype correlation between Crigler-Najjar syndrome type II and Gilbert syndrome. J Gastroenterol Hepatol 2016;31(2):403–8.

21. Bailey A, Robinson D, Dawson AM. Does Gilbert's exist? Lancet 1977;1(8018): 931–3.

22. Powell LW, Hemingway E, Billing BH, et al. Idiopathic unconjugated hyperbilirubinemia (Gilbert's syndrome). N Engl J Med 1967;277(21):1108–12.

23. Owens D, Evans J. Population studies on Gilbert's syndrome. J Med Genet 1975; 12(2):152–6.

24. Jacquemin E. Progressive familial intrahepatic cholestasis. Clin Res Hepatol Gastroenterol 2012;36(Suppl 1):S26–35.

25. Strautnieks SS, Byrne JA, Pawlikowska L, et al. Severe bile salt export pump deficiency: 82 different ABCB11 mutations in 109 families. Gastroenterology 2008; 134(4):1203–14.

26. Davit-Spraul A, Gonzales E, Baussan C, et al. Progressive familial intrahepatic cholestasis. Orphanet J Rare Dis 2009;4:1.

27. Hoerning A, Raub S, Dechene A, et al. Diversity of disorders causing neonatal cholestasis - the experience of a tertiary pediatric center in Germany. Front Pediatr 2014;2:65.

28. Fischler B, Papadogiannakis N, Nemeth A. Clinical aspects on neonatal cholestasis based on observations at a Swedish tertiary referral centre. Acta Paediatr 2001;90(2):171–8.

29. El-Guindi MA, Sira MM, Hussein MH, et al. Hepatic immunohistochemistry of bile transporters in progressive familial intrahepatic cholestasis. Ann Hepatol 2016; 15(2):222–9.

30. Davit-Spraul A, Fabre M, Branchereau S, et al. *ATP8B1* and *ABCB11* analysis in 62 children with normal gamma-glutamyl transferase progressive familial intrahepatic cholestasis (PFIC): phenotypic differences between PFIC1 and PFIC2 and natural history. Hepatology 2010;51(5):1645–55.

31. Folvik G, Hilde O, Helge GO. Benign recurrent intrahepatic cholestasis: review and long-term follow-up of five cases. Scand J Gastroenterol 2012;47(4):482–8.

32. Jung C, Driancourt C, Baussan C, et al. Prenatal molecular diagnosis of inherited cholestatic disease. J Pediatr Gastroenterol Nutr 2007;44(4):453–8.

33. Harris MJ, Le Couteur DG, Arias IM. Progressive familial intrahepatic cholestasis: genetic disorders of biliary transporters. J Gastroenterol Hepatol 2005;20(6):807–17.

34. Tygstrup N, Steig BA, Juijn JA, et al. Recurrent familial intrahepatic cholestasis in the Faeroe Islands. Phenotypic heterogeneity but genetic homogeneity. Hepatology 1999;29(2):506–8.

35. Su K, Donaldson E, Sharma R. Novel treatment options for lysosomal acid lipase deficiency: critical appraisal of sebelipase alfa. Appl Clin Genet 2016;9:157–67.

36. Bernstein DL, Hulkova H, Bialer MG, et al. Cholesteryl ester storage disease: review of the findings in 135 reported patients with an underdiagnosed disease. J Hepatol 2013;58(6):1230–43.

37. Muntoni S, Wiebusch H, Jansen-Rust M, et al. Prevalence of cholesteryl ester storage disease. Arterioscler Thromb Vasc Biol 2007;27(8):1866–8.

38. Wolman M, Sterk VV, Gatt S, et al. Primary familial xanthomatosis with involvement and calcification of the adrenals. Report of two more cases in siblings of a previously described infant. Pediatrics 1961;28:742–57.

39. Scott SA, Liu B, Nazarenko I, et al. Frequency of the cholesteryl ester storage disease common *LIPA* E8SJM mutation (c.894G>A) in various racial and ethnic groups. Hepatology 2013;58(3):958–65.

40. Pisciotta L, Fresa R, Bellocchio A, et al. Cholesteryl ester storage disease (CESD) due to novel mutations in the *LIPA* gene. Mol Genet Metab 2009;97(2):143–8.

41. Hamilton J, Jones I, Srivastava R, et al. A new method for the measurement of lysosomal acid lipase in dried blood spots using the inhibitor Lalistat 2. Clin Chim Acta 2012;413(15–16):1207–10.

42. Civallero G, de Mari J, Bittar C, et al. Extended use of a selective inhibitor of acid lipase for the diagnosis of Wolman disease and cholesteryl ester storage disease. Gene 2014;539(1):154–6.

43. Abboud RT, Nelson TN, Jung B, et al. Alpha$_1$-antitrypsin deficiency: clinical-genetic overview. Appl Clin Genet 2011;4:55–65.

44. Perlmutter DH, Brodsky JL, Balistreri WF, et al. Molecular pathogenesis of alpha-1-antitrypsin deficiency-associated liver disease: a meeting review. Hepatology 2007;45:1313–23.

45. Birrer P, McElvaney NG, Chang-Stroman LM, et al. α-1 antitrypsin deficiency and liver disease. J Inherit Metab Dis 1991;14(4):512–25.

46. Stoller JK, Aboussouan LS. A review of α1-antitrypsin deficiency. Am J Respir Crit Care Med 2012;185(3):246–59.

47. Esnault VLM, Testa A, Audrain M, et al. Alpha-1 antitrypsin genetic polymorphism in ANCA-positive systemic vasculitis. Kidney Int 1993;43(6):1329–32.

48. Smith KC, Su WPD, Pittelkow MR, et al. Clinical and pathologic correlations in 96 patients with panniculitis, including 15 patients with deficient levels of α$_1$-antitrypsin. J Am Acad Dermatol 1989;21:1192–6.

49. Hutchison DC. α$_1$-antityrspin deficiency in Europe: geographical distribution of Pi types S and Z. Respir Med 1998;92(3):367–77.

50. de Serres FJ, Blanco I. Prevalence of α1-antitrypsin deficiency alleles PI*S and PI*Z worldwide and effective screening for each of the five phenotypic classes PI*MS, PI*MZ, PI*SS, PI*SZ, and PI*ZZ: a comprehensive review. Ther Adv Respir Dis 2012;6(5):277–95.

51. Chu AS, Chopra KB, Perlmutter DH. Is severe progressive liver disease caused by alpha-1-antitrypsin deficiency more common in children or adults? Liver Transpl 2016;22(7):886–94.

52. Sveger T. Liver disease in alpha$_1$-antitrypsin deficiency detected by screening of 200,000 infants. N Engl J Med 1976;294(24):1316–21.

53. Lomas DA, Evans DL, Finch JT, et al. The mechanism of Z alpha 1-antitrypsin accumulation in the liver. Nature 1992;357(6379):605–7.

54. Eriksson S, Carlson J, Velez R. Risk of cirrhosis and primary liver cancer in alpha 1-antitrypsin deficiency. N Engl J Med 1986;314(12):736–9.

55. Hood JM, Koep LJ, Peters RL, et al. Liver transplantation for advanced liver disease with alpha-1-antitrypsin deficiency. N Engl J Med 1980;302(5):272–5.

56. Tanzi RE, Petrukhin K, Chernov I, et al. The Wilson disease gene is a copper transporting ATPase with homology to the Menkes disease gene. Nat Genet 1993;5(4):344–50.

57. Merle U, Schaefer M, Ferenci P, et al. Clinical presentation, diagnosis and long-term outcome of Wilson's disease: a cohort study. Gut 2007;56(1):115–20.

58. Roberts EA, Schilsky ML. Diagnosis and treatment of Wilson disease: an update. Hepatology 2008;47(6):2089–111.

59. Reilly M, Daly L, Hutchinson M. An epidemiological study of Wilson's disease in the Republic of Ireland. J Neurol Neurosurg Psychiatry 1993;56(3):298–300.

60. European Association for Study of Liver. EASL clinical practice guidelines: Wilson's disease. J Hepatol 2012;56(3):671–85.

61. Gow PJ, Smallwood RA, Angus PW, et al. Diagnosis of Wilson's disease: an experience over three decades. Gut 2000;446(3):415–9.

62. Sallie R, Katsiyiannakis L, Baldwin D, et al. Failure of simple biochemical indexes to reliably differentiate fulminant Wilson's disease from other causes of fulminant liver failure. Hepatology 1992;16(5):1206–11.

63. Schilsky ML, Scheinberg IH, Sternlieb I. Prognosis of Wilsonian chronic active hepatitis. Gastroenterology 1991;100(3):762–7.

64. Prashanth LK, Sinha S, Taly AB, et al. Do MRI features distinguish Wilson's disease from other early onset extrapyramidal disorders? An analysis of 100 cases. Mov Disord 2010;25(6):672–8.

65. Ferenci P, Caca K, Loudianos G, et al. Diagnosis and phenotypic classification of Wilson disease. Liver Int 2003;23(3):139–42.

66. Nicastro E, Ranucci G, Vajro P, et al. Re-evaluation of the diagnostic criteria for Wilson disease in children with mild liver disease. Hepatology 2010;52(6): 1948–56.

67. Fleming CR, Dickson ER, Wahner HW, et al. Pigmented corneal rings in non-Wilsonian liver disease. Ann Intern Med 1977;86(3):285–8.

68. Scheinberg H, Gitlin D. Deficiency of ceruloplasmin in patients with hepatolenticular degeneration. Science 1952;116(3018):4484–5.

69. Ferenci P, Steindl-Munda P, Vogel W, et al. Diagnostic value of quantitative hepatic copper determination in patients with Wilson's disease. Clin Gastroenterol Hepatol 2005;3(8):811–8.

70. Stromeyer FW, Ishak KG. Histology of the liver in Wilson's disease. Am J Clin Pathol 1980;73(1):12–24.

Liver Disease in Patients on Total Parenteral Nutrition

Arnab Mitra, MD, Joseph Ahn, MD*

KEYWORDS

- TPN • PNALD • Cholestasis of sepsis • Combined intestinal and liver failure

KEY POINTS

- Parenteral nutrition-associated liver disease (PNALD) is defined as a spectrum of liver disease ranging from abnormal liver enzymes to steatosis, to fibrosis, and eventual cirrhosis in patients on total parenteral nutrition (TPN).
- The causes of PNALD are multifactorial.
- Diagnosis of PNALD in adults is primarily by exclusion, given concomitant risk factors of critical illness and postoperative state that are present in hospitalized patients on TPN, such as sepsis, hypoxia, multiple medications, and biliary causes.
- Treatment of PNALD involves avoiding TPN if possible, or otherwise incorporating fish oil–based lipid emulsion in the TPN formulation, based on recent promising research on the latter's role in reducing risk and progression of liver disease.
- In patients with intestinal and liver failure, a combined intestine-liver transplant remains a viable option.

INTRODUCTION

Total parenteral nutrition (TPN) is defined as parenteral (intravenous [IV]) nutritional support that includes calories, amino acids, electrolytes, vitamins, minerals, and trace elements. TPN is indicated in patients for a variety of conditions revolving around intestinal insufficiency due to decreased intestine length or functionality. Most commonly, it is used in patients with short gut syndrome. Congenital causes are observed in infants born with intestinal atresia, whereas acquired causes are likely related to surgery involving small intestine resection. The latter may be in the setting of Crohn's disease or small bowel ischemia related to thrombosis, volvulus, or trauma. Functional short bowel syndrome can occur in chronic intestinal pseudo-obstruction syndrome, refractory celiac sprue disease, radiation enteritis, or congenital villous atrophy. TPN is also indicated for those with malnutrition during critical illness, and

Disclosure Statement: The authors have nothing to disclose.
Department of Medicine, Division of Gastroenterology and Hepatology, Oregon Health and Science University, 3181 Southwest Sam Jackson Park Road, L461, Portland, OR 97239-3098, USA
* Corresponding author.
E-mail address: ahnj@ohsu.edu

Clin Liver Dis 21 (2017) 687–695
http://dx.doi.org/10.1016/j.cld.2017.06.008
1089-3261/17/© 2017 Elsevier Inc. All rights reserved.

liver.theclinics.com

bowel obstruction. Studies have shown that the length of remnant intestine necessary to prevent TPN dependence is approximately 100 cm in the absence of an intact and functional colon, or approximately 50 cm in the presence of a completely functional colon.[1-2]

TPN is generally administered via central venous access, such as a peripherally inserted central catheter, port, or Hickman catheter. The need for central access stems from the toxicity of TPN to smaller peripheral veins due to the pH, osmolarity, and volume of the nutritional solution. There are several side effects and adverse effects associated with the administration of TPN. These include thrombosis of central veins and catheter-related bloodstream infections, such as fungemia, cholecystitis, and metabolic disease. This article discusses the impact of TPN on the liver and its function.

Parenteral nutrition-associated liver disease (PNALD) is a spectrum of disease that can range from mild liver enzyme abnormalities to steatosis to eventual fibrosis or cirrhosis. In general, PNALD is more prevalent in infants than in adults. In infants, especially those with low birthweight, up to 50% to 66% of those on TPN have been reported to develop PNALD.[3-6] An even higher incidence is observed in premature infants, postulated to occur because of insufficient capacity for hepatic transsulfuration, the latter being important in the metabolism of nutritional byproducts.[7-9] One study showed 65% of infants on TPN developed cholestasis and 13% eventually progressed to hepatic failure.[10] The prevalence and incidence of PNALD have not been as clearly delineated in adults as in the pediatric population. PNALD remains primarily a diagnosis of exclusion in adults on TPN.

PATHOPHYSIOLOGY

The pathophysiology of PNALD has been studied in great detail, and seems to be multifactorial in causes. The fatty acid derivatives of lipid emulsions have been shown to have an impact on systemic inflammation and oxidative stress, which can lead to liver damage.[11] It is also postulated that prolonged bowel rest with subsequent bacterial overgrowth may contribute to hepatic steatosis and cholestasis.[12,13] In patients with severe protein malnutrition, hepatic steatosis can develop because of decreased very low-density lipoprotein (VLDL) production, which results in hepatic triglyceride accumulation.[14-16]

Deficiency in choline can also result in hepatic steatosis. The proposed mechanism of this is impaired biosynthesis of choline from methionine when the latter is provided parenterally. Reversal of liver injury was seen to occur with choline supplementation within TPN solution.[14,15] Taurine deficiency is another postulated cause of PNALD, with serum levels being decreased due to cystathionase deficiency with TPN.[17-19]

Another postulated cause for the development of PNALD is toxicity from other nutrients infused in TPN. Particularly, infusion of greater than 50 kcal/kg/d of dextrose can lead to hepatic steatosis through an increase in the portal insulin or glucagon ratio.[20] Increased insulin leads to increased lipolysis and decreased hepatocyte excretion of triglycerides, in addition to inhibition of mitochondrial fatty acid oxidation, which then contributes to accumulation of fatty acids in hepatocytes.[20,21] The latter was demonstrated in a study in which glucagon was added to TPN formulation, with subsequent decrease of the insulin or glucagon ratio that prevented the development of steatosis in rats.[22,23] The lipid component in the formulation is also thought to play a role. One study determined that dosage of IV soybean oil–based lipid emulsion (SOBLE) correlates with cholestasis in children on long-term TPN, with some evidence that lipid dose greater than 1 g/kg was associated with PNALD in adults. IV fat emulsions, specifically polyunsaturated fatty acid SOBLEs are thought to be proinflammatory, containing potentially toxic phytosterols.[24] Dose and composition of IV SOBLEs have been identified as risk factors for cholestasis. It has also been postulated that the progression from hepatic steatosis to fibrosis may be related to lipid peroxidation[25] in the setting of continuous TPN.

DIAGNOSIS

Patients on TPN can develop a spectrum of abnormalities in their liver chemistries and liver disease, encompassed by the term PNALD. As previously stated, the range of disease can vary from liver enzyme abnormalities to hepatic steatosis to cholestasis to eventual fibrosis and/or cirrhosis. Clinically, PNALD is generally defined as an elevation in liver enzymes and/or alkaline phosphatase 1.5 to 3 times the upper limit of normal within 1 to 3 weeks of initiation of TPN.[7,26] It is generally uncommon for the bilirubin to increase in these first few weeks of TPN administration. In general, most patients with liver injury and/or steatosis associated with PNALD are asymptomatic. Some patients may report nonspecific abdominal discomfort related to hepatosplenomegaly.

The diagnosis of PNALD can be quite challenging due to concomitant clinical conditions that are independent risk factors for abnormal liver chemistries, as well as acute and chronic liver disease. Thus, before attributing hepatic abnormalities to TPN alone, it is critical to assess for the presence of chronic liver disease or underlying cirrhosis, in addition to other acute causes of liver injury. This applies especially to patients who are in a postoperative state or critically ill, who can have a wide range of primary diagnoses that can serve as risk factors for elevation in liver enzymes or other signs of liver disease in addition to TPN therapy.

One common cause of abnormal liver chemistries commonly seen in postoperative or critically ill patients who receive TPN is hypoxic liver injury or ischemic hepatitis. The latter may be related to circulatory shock and/or hypotension from another cause, which can be seen in the intraoperative or postoperative setting. This condition can be commonly seen in the setting of congestive heart failure or cardiogenic shock as well. Parameters, including low systemic arterial pressure, low cardiac index, low oxygen delivery, and high central venous pressure, are correlated with hepatic hypoxia and correlation with liver injury consisting of centrilobular necrosis in the setting of elevated aminotransferase levels.[21] Similar pathophysiology is associated with hypoxia and liver injury in the setting of respiratory failure.[21] The pattern of liver enzyme elevation is usually a marked increase in liver transaminases with alkaline phosphatase rarely being greater than 2 times the upper limit of normal, associated with a rapid decrease in the following days pending hemodynamic stability.

Medications related to the postoperative state can also be responsible for liver injury. These include anesthetics such as halothane, which in particular has been characterized as a primary agent that can cause liver dysfunction. Halothane is rarely used in the current clinical setting, but other anesthetics, such as methoxyflurane, enflurane, and desflurane, have also been associated with liver injury.[21] The incidence of liver injury from the latter is lower than reported with halothane.[21] Many other medications can also cause liver injury postoperatively, most commonly involving acetaminophen. However, the pattern of liver injury may be nonspecific and depend on the specific medication.

Another common clinical scenario in critically ill patients on TPN associated with abnormal liver function tests is cholestasis of sepsis. In intensive care unit (ICU) patients, sepsis is generally the most common identified cause of jaundice.[27] The liver has an important protective role in sepsis from several standpoints. It is responsible for detoxification of endotoxin or lipopolysaccharide, a key mediator in the septic process. It also is involved in the removal of bacteria from the systemic circulation, which is thought to occur through the reticuloendothelial system where Kupffer cells are active. The importance of the liver's role in defense against systemic infections may be best exemplified in the increased incidence and severity of sepsis in patient with compromised hepatic function.[21,28]

Liver dysfunction as a result of sepsis can occur as a result of 2 pathways. The first is a consequence of septic shock and hypoperfusion that can result in hepatic synthetic dysfunction, resulting in a decrease in protein synthesis and glucose levels, in addition to elevated aminotransferases. There is also a component of liver injury from the inflammatory process related to cytokine mediators, which occurs as a result of the interaction between Kupffer cells, hepatocytes, neutrophils, and endothelial cells. This can lead to secondary hepatic dysfunction with cholestasis.[21,28] Studies have suggested each episode of sepsis was found to increase the risk of PNALD by approximately 3 times.[29]

Administration of TPN can also be associated with biliary disease, including calculous and acalculous cholecystitis. This likely results from the absence of physiologic stimulatory effects of enteral fat and protein stimulation on cholecystokinin release. In critically ill patients, drainage cholecystostomy may be the sole option due to the risks of cholecystectomy. Benign postoperative intrahepatic cholestasis is also observed as a cause of postoperative jaundice that can be confused with PNALD. This is primarily diagnosed through exclusion of other causes with laboratory abnormalities primarily manifesting as elevation in serum alkaline phosphatase with aminotransferases being normal or mildly elevated. Jaundice can occur a few days after surgery and may last up to 10 days after.[21] **Box 1** lists the differential diagnosis for PNALD.

EVALUATION FOR PARENTERAL NUTRITION-ASSOCIATED LIVER DISEASE

When beginning the work-up to establish the diagnosis of PNALD, the pattern of liver chemistry abnormality proves to be very useful in guiding further tests and differential diagnosis. If transaminases are generally greater than 1000 IU/mL, the likelihood of ischemic hepatitis, viral hepatitis, or drug-induced injury is much higher compared with alternative diagnoses. If transaminases are less than 1000 IU/mL, the degree of

---

Box 1
Differential diagnosis for parenteral nutrition-associated liver disease

Hypoxic liver injury

Drug-induced liver injury (eg, anesthetics, acetaminophen)

Cholestasis of sepsis

Cholecystitis (calculous or acalculous)

Benign postoperative intrahepatic cholestasis

Chronic liver disease (eg, viral hepatitis, hemochromatosis, alpha-1 antitrypsin, nonalcoholic fatty liver disease, alcohol)

Hemolysis

Acute viral hepatitis

elevation of alkaline phosphatase and bilirubin can further help to guide whether cholestasis is present, which raises suspicion for sepsis, medications, biliary disease, or benign postoperative cholestasis. The role of imaging is quite important in this situation in helping to delineate a biliary versus nonbiliary process. The degree of bilirubin elevation and fractionation may also raise suspicion for hemolysis, which can be secondary to medications or infection, among other causes. Liver biopsy may also be a helpful adjunct in the evaluation, especially to clarify the causes of chronic liver disease or cirrhosis that may be observed for the first time. Depending on the stage of PNALD (mild, cholestatic, or with associated cirrhosis), this may be diagnosed in setting of normal or elevated bilirubin with exclusion of other aforementioned causes. **Fig. 1** presents a proposed algorithm for evaluation in this particular clinical scenario.

Treatment

The most obvious step to prevent further progression of liver disease in patients suspected of PNALD is to discontinue TPN if possible and transition to enteral nutritional support. However, this may not always be feasible, depending on the clinical circumstance of the patient, due to the persistence of severe malnutrition or unresolved anatomic or functional indications for TPN. Patients exposed to long-term TPN (defined as >6 months) may progress to steatohepatitis and micronodular cirrhosis.[7] However, if cessation of TPN occurs, reversal of cholestasis and hepatic injury can occur.[30]

There have been several studies that have delineated different types of approaches to treating PNALD. The cycling of TPN, given the periods of fasting and decreased insulin, has been postulated to help with fat mobilization and reduce hepatic steatosis.[31] Certain drugs have also been studied, including ursodiol, which has been postulated to be helpful in reducing parenteral nutrition-associated cholestasis and improving

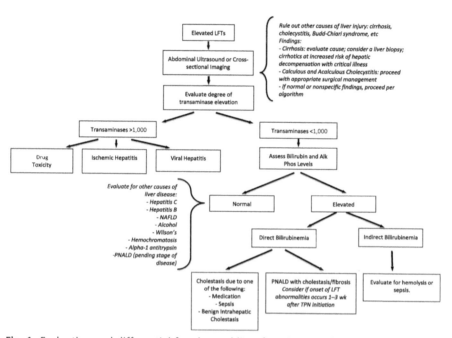

Fig. 1. Evaluation and differential for elevated liver function tests (LFTs) in the postoperative and/or critically ill patient on TPN.

overall liver function. However, prophylactic use of ursodiol in infants did not achieve this effect and ursodiol has not been recommended.[32,33] As previously discussed, dose and composition of IV SOBLE have been described as risk factors for PNALD. Studies have shown that subjects with reduced dosing of IV SOBLE overall had decreased rates of PNALD and improvement in liver chemistries.[34]

The modality that has been researched extensively and recently with demonstration of some promise is the incorporation of IV fish oil–based lipid emulsions (FOBLEs). In infants, lower death rates have been seen in those who received IV FOBLE compared with IV SOBLE.[35] Another study demonstrated reversal of PNALD in 3 out of 4 infants who had intestinal failure with the use of IV FOBLE.[36] In 9 of 12 infants with short bowel syndrome, hyperbilirubinemia associated with PNALD was reversed with a combination of IV FOBLE and SOBLE.[37]

The underlying mechanism of the relationship previously described is not completely known. Omega (n)-3 fatty acids and decreased amounts of phytosterols in IV FOBLE are postulated to have anti-inflammatory properties that may play a role in the reduced burden of PNALD.[38] In addition to these studies, which demonstrated the benefit of FOBLE in pediatric subjects, there have been recent studies that illustrate the benefit of FOBLE in adult surgical and critically ill subjects on TPN. One study showed improved liver function in subjects undergoing major abdominal surgery who received FOBLE compared with those who received SOBLE.[39] Others reported that gastrointestinal surgical subjects receiving FOBLE postoperatively reported improved liver functions compared with those receiving medium-chain triacylglycerols and long-chain triacylglycerols combination.[40] Another important study illustrated improved liver function tests in surgical and ICU subjects receiving a combination emulsion, including soybean oil, medium chain triglycerides, olive oil, and fish oil compared with those receiving purely SOBLE.[41]

More evidence supporting FOBLE comes from a recent case report of an adult with PNALD who had improvement in liver function after transition from SOBLE to FOBLE.[42] Last but not least, an additional case report showed that n-3 enriched lipid emulsion (100% fish oil) normalized TPN-induced cholestasis and resolved histochemical and ultrastructural abnormalities in an adult subject.[43] Clinically, it seems promising that FOBLE can be implemented instead of SOBLE in patients who will need long-term TPN to help reduce the risk and burden of PNALD.

In severe cases of PNALD leading to end-stage liver disease, a combined intestine-liver transplant can also be considered. Reported survival rates of intestine-liver allografts performed at 1-year and 5-year intervals were 85% and 61%, respectively.[44] Unfortunately, a large proportion of patients who are listed for combined intestine-liver transplants do not survive to transplant due to severity of illness with increased waiting-list mortality compared with other populations.[45–47] Indications for combined transplant include impending or overt liver failure, thrombosis of major central veins, frequent central line–related sepsis ($\geq$2 episodes of systemic sepsis secondary to line infection per year, $\geq$1 episode of line-related fungemia, septic shock, or acute respiratory distress syndrome). There are recent data that suggest the inclusion of a concomitant liver transplant in patients undergoing second intestinal retransplants was associated with decreased rates of intestinal rejection.[48] However, further studies are needed to refine the selection of patients for combined intestine-liver transplantation.

SUMMARY

PNALD is an important consideration in patients with abnormal liver chemistries while on TPN. The spectrum of disease ranges from steatosis to cholestasis, and eventual fibrosis pending duration of TPN and other risk factors for liver disease. The causes of PNALD are multifactorial, and potentially include possible bacterial overgrowth, decreased VLDL production in setting of malnutrition, choline deficiency, taurine deficiency, increased amount of dextrose in the formulation, and the use of SOBLEs. Hospitalized patients on TPN are commonly critically ill and/or postoperative, and, therefore, the differential diagnosis and work-up for PNALD includes evaluation for other related causes of elevated liver enzymes and underlying liver disease. To reduce the burden and progression of PNALD, transition to enteral nutrition is preferred. If not feasible, recent literature demonstrates the use of IV FOBLEs has been associated with improved liver function, reduced PNALD-related death rates, and reversal of hepatic disease progression. If end-stage liver disease develops in these clinical situations, discussion of combined intestinal-liver transplant is merited.

REFERENCES

1. Messing B, Crenn P, Beau P, et al. Long-term survival and parenteral nutrition dependence in adult patients with short bowel syndrome. Gastroenterology 1999;117:1043–50.
2. Nightingale JMD, Lennard-Jones JE, Gertner DJ, et al. Colonic preservation reduces need for parenteral therapy, increases incidence of renal stones, but does not change high prevalence of gallstones in patients with a short bowel. Gut 1992;33:1493–7.
3. Beale EF, Nelson RM, Bucciarelli RL, et al. Intrahepatic cholestasis associated with parenteral nutrition in premature infants. Pediatrics 1979;64(3):342–7.
4. Whitington PF. Cholestasis associated with total parenteral nutrition in infants. Hepatology 1985;5(4):693–6.
5. Merritt RJ. Cholestasis associated with total parenteral nutrition. J Pediatr Gastroenterol Nutr 1986;5(1):9–22.
6. Moss RL, Das JB, Raffensperger JG. Necrotizing enterocolitis and total parenteral nutrition–associated cholestasis. Nutrition 1996;12(5):340–3.
7. Buchman AL, Iyer K, Fryer J, et al. Parenteral nutrition-associated liver disease and the role for isolated intestine and intestine/liver transplantation. Hepatology 2006;43:9–19.
8. Chawla RK, Berry CJ, Kutner MH, et al. Plasma concentrations of transsulfuration pathway products during nasoenteral and intravenous hyperalimentation of malnourished patients. Am J Clin Nutr 1985;42:577–84.
9. Zlotkin SH, Anderson GH. The development of cystathionase activity during first year of life. Pediatr Res 1982;16:65–8.
10. Sondheimer JM, Asturias E, Cadnapaphornchai M. Infection and cholestasis in neonates with intestinal resection and long-term parenteral nutrition. J Pediatr Gastoenterol Nutr 1998;27:131–7.
11. Nghiem-Rao TH. Potential hepatotoxicities of intravenous fat emulsions in infants and children. Nutr Clin Pract 2016;31:619–28.
12. Pappo I, Bercovier H, Berry EM, et al. Polymyxin B reduces total parenteral nutrition-associated hepatic steatosis by its antibacterial activity and by blocking deleterious effects of lipopolysaccharide. JPEN J Parenter Enteral Nutr 1992;16(6):529–32.
13. Gupte GL, Beath SV, Kelly DA, et al. Current issues in the management of intestinal failure. Arch Dis Child 2006;91(3):259–64.
14. Buchman AL, Ament ME, Sohel M, et al. Choline deficiency causes reversible hepatic abnormalities in patients receiving parenteral nutrition: proof of a human

choline requirement: a placebo-controlled trial. JPEN J Parenter Enteral Nutr 2001;25:260–8.

15. Buchman AL, Dubin MD, Moukarzel AA, et al. Choline deficiency: a cause of hepatic steatosis during parenteral nutrition that can be reversed with intravenous choline supplementation. Hepatology 1995;22:1399–403.

16. Buchman AL, Dubin M, Jenden D, et al. Lecithin supplementation causes a decrease in hepatic steatosis in patients receiving long term parenteral nutrion. Gastroenterology 1992;102:1363–70.

17. Okamoto E, Rassin DK, Zucker CL, et al. Role of taurine in feeding the low-birth-weight infant. J Pediatr 1984;104:936–40.

18. Dorvil NP, Yousef IM, Tuchweber B, et al. Taurine prevents cholestasis induced by lithocholic acid sulfate in Guinea pigs. Am J Clin Nutr 1983;37:221–32.

19. Desai, et al. Taurine supplementation and cholestasis during bone marrow transplantation. Gastroenterology 1993;104:A616.

20. Meguid MM, Akahoshi MP, Jeffers S, et al. Amelioration of metabolic complications of conventional parenteral nutrition. Arch Surg 1984;119:1294–8.

21. Aronsohn A, Jensen D. Hepatobiliary manifestations of critically ill and postoperative patients. Clin Liver Dis 2011;15:183–97.

22. Azaz A, Thomas A, Miller V, et al. Manganese in long-term paediatric parenteral nutrition [letter]. Arch Dis Child 1995;73:89.

23. Li SJ, Nussbaum MS, McFadden DW, et al. Addition of glucagon to total parenteral nutrition (TPN) prevents hepatic steatosis in rats. Surgery 1988;104(2): 350–7.

24. Goulet O, Joly F, Corriol O, et al. Some new insights in intestinal failure–associated liver disease. Curr Opin Organ Transplant 2009;14(3):256–61.

25. MacDonald GA, Bridle KR, Ward PJ, et al. Lipid peroxidation in hepatic steatosis in humans is associated with hepatic fibrosis and occurs predominately in acinar zone 3. J Gastroenterol Hepatol 2001;16:599–606.

26. Grant JP, Cox CE, Kleinman LM, et al. Serum hepatic enzyme and bilirubin elevations during parenteral nutrition. Surg Gynecol Obstet 1977;145:573–80.

27. Whitehead MW, Hainsworth I, Kingham JG. The causes of obvious jaundice in South West Wales: perceptions versus reality. Gut 2001;48(3):409–13.

28. Gustot T, Durand F, Lebrec D, et al. Severe sepsis in cirrhosis. Hepatology 2009; 50(6):2022–33.

29. Diamond IR, de Silva NT, Tomlinson GA, et al. The role of parenteral lipids in the development of advanced intestinal failure-associated liver disease in infants: a multiple-variable analysis. JPEN J Parenter Enteral Nutr 2011;35:596–602.

30. Dahms BB, Halpin TC Jr. Serial liver biopsies in parenteral nutrition-associated cholestasis of early infancy. Gastroenterology 1981;81:136–44.

31. Chung C, Buchman AL. Postoperative jaundice and total parenteral nutrition-associated hepatic dysfunction. Clin Liver Dis 2002;6(4):1067–84.

32. Al-Hathlol K, Al-Madani A, Al-Saif S, et al. Ursodeoxycholic acid therapy for intractable total parenteral nutrition-associated cholestasis in surgical very low birth weight infants. Singapore Med J 2006;47:147–51.

33. Spagnuolo MI, Iorio R, Vegnente A, et al. Ursodeoxycholic acid for treatment of cholestasis in children on long-term total parenteral nutrition: a pilot study. Gastroenterology 1996;111:716–9.

34. Rollins MD, Ward RM, Jackson WD, et al. Effect of decreased parenteral soybean lipid emulsion on hepatic function in infants at risk for parenteral nutrition-associated liver disease. J Pediatr Surg 2013;48(6):1348–56.

35. Puder M, Valim C, Meisel JA, et al. Parenteral fish oil improves outcomes in patients with parenteral nutrition–associated liver injury. Ann Surg 2009;250(3): 395–402.
36. Cheung HM, Lam HS, Tam YH, et al. Rescue treatment of infants with intestinal failure and parenteral nutrition–associated cholestasis (PNAC) using a parenteral fish-oil-based lipid. Clin Nutr 2009;28(2):209–12.
37. Diamond IR, Sterescu A, Pencharz PB, et al. Changing the paradigm: omegaven for the treatment of liver failure in pediatric short bowel syndrome. J Pediatr Gastroenterol Nutr 2009;48(2):209–15.
38. Bharadwaj S, Gohel T, Deen OJ, et al. Fish oil-based lipid emulsion: current updates on a promising novel therapy for the management of parenteral-nutrition associated liver disease. Gastroenterol Rep (Oxf) 2015;3(2):110–4.
39. Heller AR, Rössel T, Gottschlich B, et al. Omega-3 fatty acids improve liver and pancreas function in postoperative cancer patients. Int J Cancer 2004;111: 611–6.
40. Wang J, Yu JC, Kang WM, et al. Superiority of a fish oil-enriched emulsion to medium-chain triacylglycerols/long-chain triacylglycerols in gastrointestinal surgery patients: a randomized clinical trial. Nutrition 2012;28:623–9.
41. Mertes N, Grimm H, Fürst P, et al. Safety and efficacy of a new parenteral lipid emulsion (SMOFlipid) in surgical patients: a randomized, double-blind, multi-center study. Ann Nutr Metab 2006;50:253–9.
42. Burns DL, Gill BM. Reversal of parenteral nutrition-associated liver disease with a fish oil-based lipid emulsion (Omegaven) in an adult dependent on home parenteral nutrition. JPEN J Parenter Enteral Nutr 2013;37:274–80.
43. Jurewitsch B, Gardiner G, Naccarato M, et al. Omega-3-enriched lipid emulsion for liver salvage in parenteral nutrition-induced cholestasis in the adult patient. JPEN J Parenter Enteral Nutr 2011;35:386–90.
44. Abu-Elmagd KM, Costa G, Bond GJ, et al. Five hundred intestinal and multivisceral transplantations at a single center: major advances with new challenges. Ann Surg 2009;250:567–81.
45. Fryer J, Pellar S, Ormond D, et al. Mortality in candidates waiting for combined liver-intestine transplants exceeds that for other candidates waiting for liver transplants. Liver Transpl 2003;9:748–53.
46. US Department of Health and Human Services. 2003 Annual Report. The U.S. Organ Procurement and Transplantation network and the scientific registry of transplant recipients: transplant data 1992–2002.
47. Grau T, Bonet A, Rubio M, et al. Liver dysfunction associated with artificial nutrition in critically ill patients. Crit Care 2007;11(1):R10.
48. Wu G, Cruz RJ. Liver inclusion improves outcomes of intestinal retransplantation in adults. [Corrected]. Transplantation 2015;99(8):e118.

The Liver in Oncology

Renu Dhanasekaran, MD, Paul Y. Kwo, MD*

KEYWORDS

- Drug-induced liver injury • Venooclusive liver disease
- Sinusoidal obstruction syndrome • Nodular regenerative hyperplasia
- Autoimmune hepatitis • Radiation toxicity • Hepatitis B reactivation

KEY POINTS

- Clinicians will often encounter oncologic patients with elevated liver tests or hepatic imaging abnormalities.
- Oncologic agents can cause hepatotoxicity by direct toxicity, idiosyncratic reactions, and immune-mediated hepatotoxicity.
- Those undergoing hematopoietic stem cell transplantation with preexisitng liver disease or receive certain oncologic agents are at high risk for venoocclusive disease.
- A late complication of chemotherapy can be nodular regenerative hyperplasia, with an insidious onset.
- All patients receiving chemotherapy should be screened for hepatitis B; reactivation should be considered in any patient receiving chemotherapy who presents with abnormal liver tests.

INTRODUCTION

Over the past 20 years, those who are diagnosed with solid and hematologic cancers have had an increasing number of therapeutic options to treat their malignancies. And many of these patients are experiencing improved overall survival and long-term remissions with the introduction of new classes of oncologic agents including new cytotoxic agents, targeted therapies, and immunooncologic agents. However, these new agents and combinations of agents have come with additional toxicities and, given that the liver is responsible for the metabolism of the majority of oncologic agents, hepatotoxicity may occur while receiving adjuvant therapy for a variety of solid and hematologic malignancies. Unrelated to direct hepatotoxic effects of chemotherapy to the liver, viral infections such as hepatitis B may reactivate in those who have active infection (hepatitis B surface antigen [HBsAg] positive), including those who have

Disclosure: Dr P.Y. Kwo serve on the advisory board and receives grant support from BMS and GlIead.
Department of Medicine, Stanford University School of Medicine, 750 Welch Road #210, Palo Alto, CA 94304-1507, USA
* Corresponding author.
E-mail address: pkwo@stanford.edu

Clin Liver Dis 21 (2017) 697–707
http://dx.doi.org/10.1016/j.cld.2017.06.003
1089-3261/17/© 2017 Elsevier Inc. All rights reserved.

liver.theclinics.com

cleared HBsAg.[1] The liver is also more commonly involved as an organ to which metastases spread than any other organ, including the lung, with 50% of patients with a primary malignancy developing hepatic metastases. Radiation therapy and other locoregional therapies may be used to treat metastatic lesions to the liver in addition to chemotherapy and resection. In this review, we discuss common liver-related problems encountered by those who care for patients with oncologic disorders.

CHEMOTHERAPY-INDUCED DRUG-INDUCED LIVER INJURY

Classically, drug-induced liver injury has been described as either a result of a direct hepatotoxic effect on hepatocytes (such as acetaminophen) or an idiosyncratic effect that depends on a variety of factors, including host genetic factors.[2] In general, idiosyncratic reactions are more common than direct toxic reactions (such as acetaminophen). However, many chemotherapeutic agents and regimens are dosed based on the highest dose tolerated without toxicity; thus, in oncologic patients, clinicians must recognize that both direct toxic effects of chemotherapy as well as idiosyncratic reactions can cause hepatotoxicity. In addition, preexisting liver disease may also lead to a more severe hepatotoxic pattern. That is, those with normal liver chemistries and no liver disease typically tolerate chemotherapeutic regimens better than those with advanced fibrosis or cirrhosis.[3] The presence of common hepatic disorders such as nonalcoholic fatty liver disease does not seem to increase the incidence of drug-induced liver injury, although the severity of the hepatotoxic event may be higher in the setting of chronic liver disease, particularly advanced fibrosis. Thus, many oncologic agents require dose modifications for elevations in bilirubin, aminotransferase levels, and alkaline phosphatase levels. A useful categorization of those with abnormal liver tests who have received oncologic agents is the use of the R-value. The R-value is defined as alanine aminotransferase/upper limit of normal $\div$ alkaline phosphatase/upper limit of normal. If the R-value is greater than 5, this implies hepatocellular injury; if the R-value is less than 2, this implies cholestatic injury; and if it is between 2 and 5, this implies a mixed hepatitic cholestatic pattern of injury.

Before we discuss chemotherapeutic agents that cause drug-induced liver injury, a brief review of classes of chemotherapy is in order. Cytotoxic chemotherapeutic agents may be broadly classified as alkylating agents, antimetabolites, mitotic inhibitors, and antibiotics,[4] other broad classes of chemotherapy include molecular targeted therapies and immunotherapies.

Patterns of Hepatotoxicity-Associated Oncologic Classes of Drugs

Alkylating agents
Alkylating agents are a classic group of chemotherapeutic agents that binds to DNA to prevent DNA replication. Alkylating agents are used to treat a variety of solid tumors as well as hematologic malignancies, and are generally classified as nitrogen mustards, nitrosoureas, alkyl sulfonates, triazines, and ethylenimines. As a group, the alkylating agents have low rates of hepatotoxicity with only rare reports of cholestatic hepatitis with temozolomide,[5] cyclophosphamide,[6] and chlorambucil (**Table 1**).[7]

Antimetabolites
Antimetabolites interfere with DNA replication and cell division by causing cell death when incorporated into DNA or RNA. Antimetabolites are used in the treatment of hematologic malignancies and solid tumors, including acute myelogenous leukemia, breast cancer, head and neck cancers, and gastrointestinal cancers. Hepatotoxicity has been reported with several of the antimetabolites including 6-mercaptopurine, which is used in the treatment of acute lymphoblastic leukemia, and may cause a

Table 1
Chemotherapy induced drug-induced liver injury

Class of Agent	Pattern of Hepatotoxicity	Comments
Alkylating agents: cyclophosphamide, mechlorethamine uramustine, melphalan, chlorambucil, ifosfamide, bendamustine, carmustine, lomustine, streptozocin, busulfan, cisplatin, carboplatin, nedaplatin, oxaliplatin, satraplatin, triplatin tetranitrate	Cholestatic hepatitis (mixed pattern of injury) VOD	Well-tolerated in general with low rates of hepatotoxicity Busulfan, carmustine, cyclophosphamide associated with VOD
Antimetabolites: methotrexate, 5-fluorouracil, foxuridine, cytarabine, capecitabine, and gemcitabine, 6-mercaptopurine, azathioprine, 6-thioguanine, cladribine, fludarabine, nelarabine and pentostatin	Hepatocellular pattern of injury, cholestatic pattern of injury or a mixed pattern of injury VOD	6-Mercaptopurine may cause hepatitis Azathioprine associated with NRH Methotrexate can cause steatohepatitis Cytarabine, 6-MP, azathioprine associated with VOD
Mitotic inhibitors: docetaxel, estramustine, ixabepilone, paclitaxel, vinblastine, vincristine, vinorelbine	Hepatocellular pattern of injury	Typically well-tolerated with only rare cases of clinically significant hepatotoxicity
Topoisomerase inhibitors: irinotecan, topotecan, camptothecin lamellarin D, etoposide (VP-16), teniposide, doxorubicin, daunorubicin, mitoxantrone, mitomycin, bleomycin, dactinomycin, plicamycin, amsacrine	Hepatocellular pattern of the injury, cholestatic pattern of injury or a mixed pattern of injury	Plicamycin associated with severe hepatotoxicity Irinotecan can be associated with severe side effects in those who carry the UGT1A1*28
Molecular targeted therapies: erlotinib, gefitnib, imatinib, ipilimumab, tremelimumab, nivolumab, pembrolizumab, gemtuzumab ozogamicin	Hepatocellular pattern of injury, jaundice, VOD	Gemtuzumab ozogamicin implicated in VOD Ipilimumab and tremelimumab with higher rates of immune hepatitis Erlotinib, gefitnib with jaundice

Abbreviations: 6-MP, 6-mercaptopurine; NRH, nodular regenerative hyperplasia; VOD, venoocclusive disease.

hepatocellular pattern of the injury, a cholestatic pattern of injury, or a mixed pattern of injury.[8,9] Azathioprine is a derivative of 6-mercaptopurine and may also cause hepatotoxicity, although at lower rates than 6-mercaptopurine. Azathioprine is also associated with nodular regenerative hyperplasia.[10] Methotrexate is an antimetabolite that has been implicated in multiple forms of hepatic injury, including steatohepatitis with fibrosis and cirrhosis, as well as a hepatocellular pattern of injury. Similarly, tamoxifen, an estrogen receptor blocker commonly used in the treatment of estrogen receptor–positive breast cancer, is associated with the development of nonalcoholic fatty liver disease and nonalcoholic steatohepatitis.[11]

Mitotic inhibitors

The mitotic inhibitors include spindle inhibitors, topoisomerase inhibitors, and platinums. The spindle inhibitors include vincristine, paclitaxel, and docetaxel, and are used to treat a variety of solid tumors including lung cancer. They have been associated with elevated liver tests when used in combination with radiation therapy, although these increase rarely cause clinically significant liver injury.[12,13] In addition, dose reductions are required in those with hepatic impairment or elevated liver tests.[14] However, significant hepatotoxicity is rare with this class of medicine. Topoisomerase inhibitors have been reported to cause hepatocellular, cholestatic, and mixed patterns of injury. One of the topoisomerase inhibitors, irinotecan, which is used in a variety of solid tumors, including colorectal, ovarian, and lung cancers, is associated with particularly severe side effects in those who carry the UGT1A1*28 polymorphism.[15] The platinum class including cisplatin and carboplatin typically cause minor increases in aminotransferase levels with rare cases of significant hepatotoxicity.

Antitumor antibiotics

Antitumor antibiotics are used in the treatment of hematologic and solid tumors, and include bleomycin, dactinomycin, daunorubicin, doxorubicin, mitomycin, mitoxantrone, plicamycin. They are associated with a low level of hepatotoxicity except for plicamycin, which can lead to marked elevations in aspartate aminotransferase (AST) and alanine aminotransferase (ALT) levels and is thus a rarely used chemotherapeutic agent.[4] Many of the antitumor antibiotic agents are associated with the development of venoocclusive disease (VOD) and sinusoidal obstruction syndrome (SOS).

Molecular targeted therapies

The other class of oncologic agents that may lead to hepatotoxicity is the molecular targeted therapies that include monoclonal antibodies and small molecule oral kinase inhibitors. These agents block pathways involved in tumor progression, angiogenesis, tissue invasion, metastasis, immune response, and many other biological processes, and have revolutionized the treatment of solid tumors. However, side effects do occur; many of these molecular targets are also expressed in normal tissues. The epidermal growth factor receptor tyrosine kinase inhibitors erlotinib and gefitnib, which are used for treatment of non–small cell lung cancer, are associated with hyperbilirubinemia owing to uridine gluconuryl transferase inhibition.[16–18] Severe hepatic injury has been reported in patients with underlying liver disease who received these drugs and hence close monitoring is required in those with moderate to severe hepatic dysfunction.[19] The tyrosine kinase inhibitor imatinib is an effective therapy for chronic myelogenous leukemia, but has been associated with significant increases in AST and ALT in those with advanced disease. The increases typically resolve after discontinuation of imatinib.[20] Lapatanib is a dual inhibitor of human epidermal growth factor receptor 2, neu, and the epidermal growth factor receptor, and has been reported to be associated with severe hepatotoxicity and patients receiving this agent require weekly monitoring of liver enzymes.[21] Similarly pazopanib, an oral multikinase inhibitor, has led to severe hepatotoxicity and genome-wide association studies have revealed that HLA-B*57:01 confers susceptibility for hepatotoxicity.[22] More important, sorafenib and regorafenib, 2 multikinase inhibitors approved for the treatment of hepatocellular carcinoma, are themselves associated with hepatotoxicity and need to be discontinued if grade 3 AST and ALT elevations occur.[23] Finally, the targeted therapy gemtuzumab ozogamicin has been associated with VOD with SOS.[24]

Immunotherapy

Immunooncologic agents work by targeting pathways that prevent overactivation of cytotoxic T cells like programmed death receptors cytotoxic T-lymphocyte–associated protein 4 (CTLA-4) and programmed cell death-1 (PD-1) and restore immune-mediated antitumor activity.[25] However, owing to their mechanism, immune-mediated hepatic injury occurs as part of the immune-mediated adverse event profile. A recent large review found that CTLA-4 inhibitors (ipilimumab and tremelimumab) were associated with a higher rate of all-grade and high-grade hepatotoxicity compared with the PD-1 inhibitors (nivolumab and pembrolizumab) with an onset of 6 to 14 weeks.[26] The rate of hepatotoxicity with CTLA-4 blockade alone is less than 10%,[27] but it can increase to up to 20% with blockade of both CTLA-4 and PD-1. These individuals with high AST and ALT levels are managed like those with autoimmune hepatitis, with corticosteroids and other adjunctive immunosuppressive agents. Mycophenolate mofetil can be used for the management of steroid-unresponsive cases.

VENOOCCLUSIVE DISEASE AND SINUSOIDAL OBSTRUCTION SYNDROME

VOD and SOS is a unique disorder that occurs after bone marrow transplant, typically myeloablative hematopoietic stem cell transplantation. VOD with SOS is believed to be a consequence high-dose chemotherapy involving agents primarily metabolized by the liver including alkylating agents, antimetabolites, and combination of agents administered before transplantation, which are toxic to sinusoidal endothelial cells and hepatocytes.[28] The incidence of hematopoietic stem cell transplantation varies between 0% and 40% with a recent large review suggesting an overall incidence of 13.7%.[29] Pretransplant risk factors include underlying liver disease, age, and administration of certain chemotherapeutic agents (anti-CD33 monoclonal antibody gemtuzumab, ozogamicin) before transplantation. Transplantation-related risk factors include busulphan and cyclophosphamide administration as well as the use of high-dose radiation. The clinical presentation of VOD is typically within 30 days of transplantation, with patients developing ascites fluid retention with weight gain, jaundice, and symptomatic hepatomegaly, and the diagnosis can be made on clinical grounds. These clinical findings are accompanied by changes in laboratory tests, including elevations in aminotransferase levels, bilirubin, prothrombin time, and reduced albumin. A helpful rule of thumb has been a bilirubin level of 20 mg/dL at day 20 portends a poor prognosis.

A Doppler ultrasound examination of the liver may demonstrate reversal of flow in the portal vein, ascites, or changes in the hepatic artery resistive index, but none are diagnostic of VOD. Although not required for the diagnosis, in cases where the diagnosis of VOD is not clear, transjugular liver biopsy with pressure measurement demonstrating hepatic vein pressure gradient of greater than 10 mm has a high sensitivity and specificity. The clinical course of VOD is determined by the clinical severity. The majority of cases of VOD are mild cases where the bilirubin level remains below 3 mg/dL, the disease is self-limited, and full recovery is expected. Moderate cases require a longer time to recover with bilirubin levels of up to 5 mg/dL, aminotransferase levels up to 5 times the upper limit of normal, and development of weight gain and acute kidney injury. These individuals may require close follow-up. Similar to those with mild VOD, those with moderate disease can be supported with diuretics and analgesics for their edema, infiltrates, and ascites, and most recover. Those with severe VOD have a more rapidly progressive course with bilirubin levels increasing above 5 mg/dL and development of multisystem organ failure and high mortality rates of greater than 90%. No prophylactic therapies have been shown to be beneficial, although they have been studied extensively.

The recent approval of defibrotide, a compound consisting of single-stranded polydeoxyribonucleotide sodium salts that serves to protect the endothelial cells by restoring thrombofinbrinolytic balance, for severe VOD has been a welcome addition to our therapeutic armamentarium. Phase III trials have demonstrated the efficacy of defibrotide in those who developed severe VOD with multiorgan dysfunction after hematopoietic stem cell transplantation and was associated with a significant improvement of day +100 survival after hematopoietic stem cell transplantation of 38.2% versus 25.0% in the historical control group.[30,31] Defibrotide is currently approved in the United States for VOD and SOS with evidence of renal or pulmonary dysfunction.

NODULAR REGENERATIVE HYPERPLASIA

Nodular regenerative hyperplasia or noncirrhotic portal hypertension is a sequelae of multiple chemotherapeutic agents. The exact mechanism is not known but it is believed that local ischemia leads to a microscopic obliterative portal venopathy with compensatory hyperplasia of adjacent hepatocytes, leading to complications of portal hypertension without fibrosis.[32] Multiple oncologic agents have been reported to cause nodular regenerative hyperplasia and the diagnosis must be considered in those presenting with elevated liver tests as well as complications of portal hypertension. The diagnosis of nodular regenerative hyperplasia is challenging because there can be a relatively long period between the development of clinical symptoms and drug exposure, although this period (called the latency period) seems in general to be shorter with oncologic agents.[33] There is no specific pattern of liver test abnormality with elevations of AST, ALT, alkaline phosphatase, and bilirubin occurring. Imaging may show small nodules, but often is not helpful. The diagnosis rests on a high index of suspicion and transjugular liver biopsy with pressure measurements. Because of the subtle findings, a wedge biopsy may be required to appreciate the subtle architectural findings. Treatment is directed toward the complications of portal hypertension, including diuretics.[34]

HEPATITIS B REACTIVATION

Hepatitis B reactivation may occur in HBsAg-positive, and HBsAg-negative and anti-hepatitis B core antigen–positive individuals receiving a broad range of chemotherapeutic agents, with a clinical presentation ranging from mild aminotransferase elevations to acute liver failure (**Table 2**). The risk of reactivation depends on the serologic status of the patient as well as the type of chemotherapy. As an example, B-cell–depleting agents such as rituximab and ofatumumab may lead to hepatitis B reactivation in those who are HBsAg negative/anti-hepatitis B core antigen positive. But the majority of other oncologic agents will not increase the risk of reactivation in the HBsAg negative patient, but rather reactivation occurs in HBsAg-positive individuals who receive chemotherapy from classes such as the anthracyclines.[35] A recent guideline recommended routine prophylaxis in high-risk individuals and suggested prophylaxis in moderate risk individuals.[1] Regardless, all patients who are undergoing chemotherapy should be screened for hepatitis B with HBsAg and anti-hepatitis B core antigen. The presence of anti-HBsAg should not be used to decide for or against the use of prophylaxis with nucleotide and nucleoside analogues. Prophylactic therapy with tenofovir or entecavir is typically continued for 6 to 12 months after the discontinuation of chemotherapy.

Table 2
Classes of agents that can lead to hepatitis B reactivation

Class	Agents
Corticosteroids	Dexamethasone, methylprednisolone, prednisolone
Antitumor antibiotics	Actinomycin D, bleomycin, daunorubicin, doxorubicin, epirubicin, mitomycin C
Plant alkaloids	Vinblastine, vincristine
Alkylating agents	Carboplatin, chlorambucil, cisplatin, cyclophosphamide, ifosfamide
Antimetabolites	Azauridine, cytarabine, fluoracil, gemcitabine, mercaptopurine, methotrexate, thioguanine
Monoclonal antibodies	Alemtuzumab, rituximab, infliximab
Others	Colaspase, docetaxel, etoposide, fludarabine, folinic acid, interferon, procarbazine

METASTATIC LESIONS TO THE LIVER

The liver is involved in solid tumor metastases more commonly than any other organ. Even tumors from organs that do not drain into the liver via the portal circulation such as breast and lung often present with metastases to the liver, although this is typically in a pattern of disseminated metastatic disease.[36] Colorectal cancer and neuroendocrine tumors often present a single hepatic metastasis. The diagnosis is suggested by axial imaging, typically computed tomography scan with contrast and in combination with fluorodeoxyglucose-positron emission tomography scanning.[37]

Patients presenting with an isolated metastasis from colorectal cancer should be presented to a multidisciplinary committee and there are 3 strategies that historically have been used. The most common strategy has been to resect the primary cancer (with radiation if rectal cancer is the primary), then administer adjuvant chemotherapy followed by hepatic resection 3 to 6 months later. The second strategy has been to simultaneously resect the primary colorectal cancer and hepatic lesion in combination with neoadjuvant or adjuvant chemotherapy. The third option that has been proposed is to resect the primary hepatic lesion first, then give chemotherapy, then resect the primary lesion if there is not a risk of obstruction or perforation. Other ablative techniques may be used in place of surgery, such as radiofrequency ablation or stereotactic radiation in those who are poor surgical candidates or where liver remnant concerns exist.[38] A recent review suggested that all 3 approaches may be used and that none are inferior to other approaches.[39]

Neuroendocrine tumors also present with isolated hepatic metastases. Typically the primary is in the gastrointestinal tract, although the primary may originate from a pulmonary source.[40,41] The presentation may be one of synchronous metastasis or subsequent metastatic presentation. Neuroendocrine tumors typically have a less aggressive course than other solid tumors and, thus management may conservative, although surgical resection of metastatic lesions may be associated with improved survival of up to 85% in certain series of patients. Moreover, other locoregional therapies may also be used, including stereotactic radiation and radiofrequency ablation. Finally, orthotopic liver transplantation has rarely been used in more extensive disease with acceptable long-term outcomes and, recently, multivisceral transplantation with abdominal exenteration has been proposed as a method to reduce the incidence of recurrence.[41,42]

RADIATION-INDUCED LIVER INJURY

Radiation therapy is often used to treat lesions in the liver with recognition of stereo-tactic body radiation therapy as an effective treatment of primary and metastatic hepatic lesions. Radiation-induced liver disease is a well-described cause of liver injury that occurs in the first 4 months after conventional external beam radiation ther-apy. With stereotactic body radiation therapy, radiation injury can be minimized by limiting the total dose of radiation to 40 Gy for patients with cirrhosis and 70 Gy in pa-tients without cirrhosis.[43] The pattern of injury is variable, ranging from a VOD with SOS–type syndrome with ascites, hepatomegaly, and an elevated alkaline phospha-tase to a pattern of hepatocellular injury typically occurring within 3 to 4 months of treatment. The treatment is supportive.

The advent of radioembolization with the delivery of yttrium-90–coated micro-spheres to multiple segments of the liver has allowed radiologists to treat multiple tumors owing to their preferential arterial blood supply. Although the majority of the yttrium-90 is directed to the tumor, some radiation is delivered to the non–tumor-con-taining liver, leading to a syndrome of radioembolization-induced liver disease.[44] In patients with cirrhosis, those with elevated bilirubin greater than 1.2 mg/dL and small liver volume (<1.5 L) are at greater risk for radioembolization-induced liver disease where patients present within 2 months of radioembolization with jaundice and ascites but without tumor progression. In those without cirrhosis who have metastatic tumors, prior treatment with chemotherapy seems to increase the risk of radioembolization-induced liver disease.

SUMMARY

Oncologic patients can develop liver test abnormalities owing to various reasons—namely, drug toxicities from chemotherapy, occurrence of primary or secondary hepat-ic malignancies, de novo development of acute or chronic liver disease as a sequelae of chemotherapy, reactivation of hepatitis B, or radiation-induced liver injury. Chemotherapy-induced drug-induced liver injury can result both from direct toxic ef-fects, as well as from idiosyncratic patterns of injury and may be associated with unique patterns of liver injury including VOD with SOS or nodular regenerative hyperplasia. The arrival of immunotherapies has ushered in an exciting era in cancer treatment, but these oncologic agents can lead to autoimmune hepatitis–like liver injury that need to be treated with drug discontinuation and corticosteroids. Another important complication of chemotherapy can be reactivation of hepatitis B; hence, all these patients should be tested for hepatitis B before initiation of chemotherapy. Finally, management of metas-tases to the liver needs to determined based on the site of the primary and the resect-ability of the metastatic lesion. Oncologists, gastroenterologists, and hepatologists who take care of patients with cancer need to be aware of these liver-related compli-cations to make an early diagnosis and initiate appropriate treatment.

REFERENCES

1. Reddy KR, Beavers KL, Hammond SP, et al. American Gastroenterological Asso-ciation Institute guideline on the prevention and treatment of hepatitis B virus re-activation during immunosuppressive drug therapy. Gastroenterology 2015; 148(1):215–9 [quiz: e16–7].

2. Chalasani NP, Hayashi PH, Bonkovsky HL, et al. ACG clinical guideline: the diag-nosis and management of idiosyncratic drug-induced liver injury. Am J Gastroen-terol 2014;109(7):950–66.

3. Chalasani N, Regev A. Drug-induced liver injury in patients with preexisting chronic liver disease in drug development: how to identify and manage? Gastroenterology 2016;151(6):1046–51.

4. King PD, Perry MC. Hepatotoxicity of chemotherapy. Oncologist 2001;6(2):162–76.

5. Dixit S, Baker L, Walmsley V, et al. Temozolomide-related idiosyncratic and other uncommon toxicities: a systematic review. Anticancer Drugs 2012;23(10):1099–106.

6. Goldberg JW, Lidsky MD. Cyclophosphamide-associated hepatotoxicity. South Med J 1985;78(2):222–3.

7. Grigorian A, O'Brien CB. Hepatotoxicity secondary to chemotherapy. J Clin Transl Hepatol 2014;2(2):95–102.

8. Shorey J, Schenker S, Suki WN, et al. Hepatotoxicity of mercaptopurine. Arch Intern Med 1968;122(1):54–8.

9. Present DH, Meltzer SJ, Krumholz MP, et al. 6-Mercaptopurine in the management of inflammatory bowel disease: short- and long-term toxicity. Ann Intern Med 1989;111(8):641–9.

10. Barrowman JA, Kutty PK, Ra MU, et al. Sclerosing hepatitis and azathioprine. Dig Dis Sci 1986;31(2):221–2.

11. Pratt DS, Knox TA, Erban J. Tamoxifen-induced steatohepatitis [3]. Ann Intern Med 1995;123(3):236.

12. el Saghir NS, Hawkins KA. Hepatotoxicity following vincristine therapy. Cancer 1984;54(9):2006–8.

13. Hohneker JA. A summary of vinorelbine (Navelbine) safety data from North American clinical trials. Semin Oncol 1994;21(5 Suppl 10):42–6 [discussion: 6–7].

14. Floyd J, Mirza I, Sachs B, et al. Hepatotoxicity of chemotherapy. Semin Oncol 2006;33(1):50–67.

15. Raymond E, Boige V, Faivre S, et al. Dosage adjustment and pharmacokinetic profile of irinotecan in cancer patients with hepatic dysfunction. J Clin Oncol 2002;20(21):4303–12.

16. Ghatalia P, Je Y, Mouallem NE, et al. Hepatotoxicity with vascular endothelial growth factor receptor tyrosine kinase inhibitors: a meta-analysis of randomized clinical trials. Crit Rev Oncol Hematol 2015;93(3):257–76.

17. Huang YS, An SJ, Chen ZH, et al. Three cases of severe hepatic impairment caused by erlotinib. Br J Clin Pharmacol 2009;68(3):464–7.

18. Sanford M, Scott LJ. Gefitinib: a review of its use in the treatment of locally advanced/metastatic non-small cell lung cancer. Drugs 2009;69(16):2303–28.

19. Liu W, Makrauer FL, Qamar AA, et al. Fulminant hepatic failure secondary to erlotinib. Clin Gastroenterol Hepatol 2007;5(8):917–20.

20. Sawyers CL, Hochhaus A, Feldman E, et al. Imatinib induces hematologic and cytogenetic responses in patients with chronic myelogenous leukemia in myeloid blast crisis: results of a phase II study. Blood 2002;99(10):3530–9.

21. Azim HA Jr, Agbor-Tarh D, Bradbury I, et al. Pattern of rash, diarrhea, and hepatic toxicities secondary to lapatinib and their association with age and response to neoadjuvant therapy: analysis from the NeoALTTO trial. J Clin Oncol 2013;31(36):4504–11.

22. Xu CF, Johnson T, Wang X, et al. HLA-B*57:01 confers susceptibility to pazopanib-associated liver injury in patients with cancer. Clin Cancer Res 2016;22(6):1371–7.

23. Miller AA, Murry DJ, Owzar K, et al. Phase I and pharmacokinetic study of sorafenib in patients with hepatic or renal dysfunction: CALGB 60301. J Clin Oncol 2009;27(11):1800–5.

24. Nabhan C, Rundhaugen L, Jatoi M, et al. Gemtuzumab ozogamicin (MylotargTM) is infrequently associated with sinusoidal obstructive syndrome/veno-occlusive disease. Ann Oncol 2004;15(8):1231–6.

25. Loriot Y, Perlemuter G, Malka D, et al. Drug insight: gastrointestinal and hepatic adverse effects of molecular-targeted agents in cancer therapy. Nat Clin Pract Oncol 2008;5(5):268–78.

26. Wang W, Lie P, Guo M, et al. Risk of hepatotoxicity in cancer patients Treated with immune checkpoint inhibitors: a systematic review and meta-analysis of published data. Int J Cancer 2017. [Epub ahead of print].

27. Bernardo SG, Moskalenko M, Pan M, et al. Elevated rates of transaminitis during ipilimumab therapy for metastatic melanoma. Melanoma Res 2013;23(1):47–54.

28. Dalle JH, Giralt SA. Hepatic veno-occlusive disease after hematopoietic stem cell transplantation: risk factors and stratification, prophylaxis, and treatment. Biol Blood Marrow Transplant 2016;22(3):400–9.

29. Coppell JA, Richardson PG, Soiffer R, et al. Hepatic veno-occlusive disease following stem cell transplantation: incidence, clinical course, and outcome. Biol Blood Marrow Transplant 2010;16(2):157–68.

30. Richardson PG, Riches ML, Kernan NA, et al. Phase 3 trial of defibrotide for the treatment of severe veno-occlusive disease and multi-organ failure. Blood 2016; 127(13):1656–65.

31. Richardson PG, Smith AR, Triplett BM, et al. Defibrotide for patients with hepatic veno-occlusive disease/sinusoidal obstruction syndrome: interim results from a treatment IND study. Biol Blood Marrow Transplant 2017;23(6):997–1004.

32. Wanless IR. Micronodular transformation (nodular regenerative hyperplasia) of the liver: a report of 64 cases among 2,500 autopsies and a new classification of benign hepatocellular nodules. Hepatology 1990;11(5):787–97.

33. Ghabril M, Vuppalanchi R. Drug-induced nodular regenerative hyperplasia. Semin Liver Dis 2014;34(2):240–5.

34. Khanna R, Sarin SK. Non-cirrhotic portal hypertension - diagnosis and management. J Hepatol 2014;60(2):421–41.

35. Yeo W, Chan TC, Leung NWY, et al. Hepatitis B virus reactivation in lymphoma patients with prior resolved hepatitis B undergoing anticancer therapy with or without rituximab. J Clin Oncol 2009;27(4):605–11.

36. Choti MA, Bulkley GB. Management of hepatic metastases. Liver Transpl Surg 1999;5(1):65–80.

37. Page AJ, Weiss MJ, Pawlik TM. Surgical management of noncolorectal cancer liver metastases. Cancer 2014;120(20):3111–21.

38. Nordlinger B, Van Cutsem E, Gruenberger T, et al. Combination of surgery and chemotherapy and the role of targeted agents in the treatment of patients with colorectal liver metastases: recommendations from an expert panel. Ann Oncol 2009;20(6):985–92.

39. Lykoudis PM, O'Reilly D, Nastos K, et al. Systematic review of surgical management of synchronous colorectal liver metastases. Br J Surg 2014;101(6):605–12.

40. Frilling A, Modlin IM, Kidd M, et al. Recommendations for management of patients with neuroendocrine liver metastases. Lancet Oncol 2014;15(1):e8–21.

41. Florman S, Toure B, Kim L, et al. Liver transplantation for neuroendocrine tumors. J Gastrointest Surg 2004;8(2):208–12.

42. Mangus RS, Tector AJ, Kubal CA, et al. Multivisceral transplantation: expanding indications and improving outcomes. J Gastrointest Surg 2013;17(1):179–87.

43. Doi H, Shiomi H, Masai N, et al. Threshold doses and prediction of visually apparent liver dysfunction after stereotactic body radiation therapy in cirrhotic and normal livers using magnetic resonance imaging. J Radiat Res 2016;57(3): 294–300.

44. Gil-Alzugaray B, Chopitea A, Iñarrairaegui M, et al. Prognostic factors and prevention of radioembolization-induced liver disease. Hepatology 2013;57(3): 1078–87.

An Update on the Treatment and Follow-up of Patients with Primary Biliary Cholangitis

 CrossMark

Blaire E. Burman, MD[a], Manan A. Jhaveri, MD, MPH[b],
Kris V. Kowdley, MD[b,*]

KEYWORDS

- Primary biliary cholangitis • Cholestasis • Cirrhosis • Fatigue • Pruritus

KEY POINTS

- Primary biliary cholangitis (PBC) is an increasingly recognized chronic liver disease with variable presentation and prognosis.
- Without treatment, PBC is often progressive toward cirrhosis and its complications; however, survival has improved significantly with earlier diagnosis and introduction of effective therapies.
- Comorbid symptoms and conditions have a significant impact on quality of life for patients with PBC and should be managed independent of underlying liver disease.

EPIDEMIOLOGY

Although rare, primary biliary cholangitis (PBC) remains the most common chronic cholestatic liver disease among adults in the United States, with prevalence ranging from 1.91 to 40.2 per 100,000 per year, although accurate population-based data are lacking.[1] The prevalence of PBC varies worldwide, but is highest in northern Europe and North America. Such geographic variability implies a role of environmental triggers in pathogenesis, and familial clustering of PBC suggests genetic susceptibility. Interestingly, the prevalence seems to be increasing, although whether this is related to a higher case detection rate or a true increase in the burden of disease is unknown.[2] Women are disproportionately affected at a ratio of approximately 10:1, and most patients are diagnosed in the fourth or fifth decade of life.[3]

[a] Division of Gastroenterology and Hepatology, Virginia Mason Medical Center, 1100 Ninth Avenue, Seattle, WA 98101, USA; [b] Department of Organ Transplant & Liver Center, Liver Care Network and Organ Care Research, Swedish Medical Center, Seattle, 1124 Columbia Street, WA 98101, USA
* Corresponding author. 1124 Columbia Street, Suite 600, Seattle, WA 98104.
E-mail address: kris.kowdley@swedish.org

Clin Liver Dis 21 (2017) 709–723
http://dx.doi.org/10.1016/j.cld.2017.06.005
1089-3261/17/© 2017 Elsevier Inc. All rights reserved.

liver.theclinics.com

PATHOGENESIS

The pathogenesis of PBC is complex and multifaceted, and remains incompletely characterized. PBC is thought to result from an aberrant autoimmune response to environmental exposures in genetically susceptible individuals. Whereas target mitochondrial antigens are present in all body cells, the immune attack in PBC seems to be highly specific for the biliary epithelium.[4] Persistent innate and adaptive immune responses to intralobular bile ducts generate chronic inflammation that leads to destruction and loss of bile ducts and cholestasis. In turn, chronic cholestasis leads to an accumulation of intrahepatic (and systemic) cytotoxic bile acids that perpetuate liver cell injury and death.[5,6]

PBC has been associated with environmental triggers including geographic proximity to toxic waste disposal (ie, Superfund sites) and low-income areas with higher rates of pollution and cigarette smoking, in addition to household chemicals (nail polish, hair dyes), and various infectious agents.[7,8] A true causative link between 1 or more environmental triggers and PBC, however, has not been established. There is clearly a genetic component to PBC pathogenesis, and the prevalence of PBC in families with 1 affected member is 100-fold greater than the general population.[9] Multiple different immune pathways are affected including those involved in cell differentiation, antigen presentation, T-cell differentiation, and B-cell function. It has been suggested that an important component of immunologic tolerance depends on genes located on the X chromosome and may explain the reason that the vast majority of patients with PBC are women.[10]

NATURAL HISTORY

PBC was previously a leading indication for liver transplantation, and most patients were diagnosed at advanced stages of disease. The classical presentation of PBC is in middle-aged, typically postmenopausal women, with a median survival historically approximately 10 years from the diagnosis in patients with advanced disease.[11] In the era when liver biopsy was performed to establish the diagnosis and without effective therapy, the median time to develop extensive fibrosis was approximately 2 years.[12] However, with the advent of highly accurate antimitochondrial antibodies for the diagnosis of PBC, the diagnosis is increasingly made among younger patients and at an early precirrhotic stage. Currently, 60% of patients are asymptomatic at the time of diagnosis, although only 5% will remain symptom free over time.[3]

The natural history of PBC has changed in the past 2 decades owing to earlier diagnosis and the introduction of effective treatment with ursodeoxycholic acid (UDCA). The availability of UDCA has led to substantial improvements in patient outcomes. UDCA delays or prevents histologic progression of the disease and reduces the risk of esophageal varices, decompensated liver disease, need for liver transplantation, and mortality.[13,14] Survival for those who have a biochemical response to UDCA is similar to that of age-matched healthy controls.[15] UDCA lowers the progression rate from early stage disease to advanced fibrosis or cirrhosis as compared with placebo. A large metaanalysis of patients and subsequent long-term cohort studies cited an overall transplant-free survival of 90% at 5 years, 78% at 10 years, and 66% at 15 years for UDCA-treated patients as compared with 79% at 5 years, 59% at 10 years, and 32% at 15 years for untreated patients with PBC.[13,16] Sixteen percent of patients treated with UDCA developed varices as compared with 58% who received placebo with no difference in the rate of bleeding between the 2 groups.[13]

Biochemical response to UDCA is an important predictor of disease prognosis. Of the approximately 40% of patients with PBC who do not respond or are intolerant to

UDCA, the majority have more rapid disease progression and higher relative risk of death or liver transplant,[16,17] particularly those with elevated bilirubin levels. Younger age at presentation and male sex are important predictors of nonresponse to UDCA.[18]

PROGNOSTIC MODELS

Multiple prognostic models have been developed to predict the probability of survival in PBC. These models have used clinical, biochemical, and histologic parameters. Various studies have identified age at the time of diagnosis, presence of hepatomegaly, increased serum bilirubin levels, albumin, ascites, and portal fibrosis as independent predictors of survival.[19–22] The European Model[19] and the Mayo Risk Score[21] were the most frequently used models until the recent establishment of the GLOBE score.

The Mayo Risk Model was published in 1989 and validated in multiple independent cohorts.[21] It included only clinical and biochemical variables without any histologic parameters. Variables included were age of the patient, bilirubin, albumin, prothrombin time, and severity of edema. Because this model was based on baseline characteristics of patients, it was not useful to predict survival over time. van Dam and colleagues[23] developed an adapted Mayo model using the same variables to predict short-term survival or time to transplantation at any time point during repeated follow-up visits. Angulo and colleagues[24] demonstrated that the Mayo risk score was an independent risk factor predictive of development of varices ($P<.01$). The authors found that 93% of patients who developed varices had a Mayo risk score of greater than or equal to 4.[24] Corpechot and colleagues[25] proposed a Markov model to study the effect of UDCA on the natural history of disease in patients treated with 13 to 15 mg/kg/d. The overall survival rates without liver transplantation were 84% and 66% at l0 and 20 years, respectively. The survival rate was better than the spontaneous survival rate as predicted by the updated Mayo model ($P<.01$).

Because most predictive models for risk stratification of patients with PBC are based on data from a single center, the Global PBC Study Group established the PBC GLOBE score to represent a more generalizable predictive model. It is based on data from multiple international cohorts of more than 4500 patients with PBC that examined the transplant-free survival of patients receiving UDCA therapy. The GLOBE score formulated the risk of liver transplantation or death as a function of serum alkaline phosphatase (ALP) and total bilirubin after 1 year of UDCA treatment.[26] The PBC GLOBE score incorporates age at the time of initiating UDCA therapy, serum ALP, total bilirubin, albumin, and platelet counts. Lammers and colleagues[16] conducted a metaanalysis to evaluate the impact of serum ALP and total bilirubin levels on long-term outcomes such as liver transplantation and death. The authors concluded that the 10-year survival rate without a liver transplant after 1 year of treatment with UDCA was 84% in patients with an ALP level of twice the upper limit of normal and 86% with bilirubin levels of less than or equal to two times the upper limit of normal as compared with 62% in patients with ALP level of less than twice the upper limit of normal ($P<.0001$) and 41% with bilirubin levels greater than the upper limit of normal ($P<.0001$).[16]

DIAGNOSIS

Most patients with PBC are diagnosed when routine blood work reveals abnormal liver enzymes and leading to subsequent evaluation, often before the onset of symptoms. ALP elevations are predominant over hepatocellular liver enzyme elevations. Although aspartate aminotransferase (AST) and alanine aminotransferase may be increased in

PBC, overlap with autoimmune hepatitis should be considered when greater than 5-fold normal.[3] Total and direct bilirubin levels are usually normal in early stage disease, although these become elevated as the disease progresses and predict worse prognosis.[21] The combination of ALP at least 1.5 times the upper limit of normal and presence of antimitochondrial antibody (AMA) at a titer of 1:40 or higher can be considered diagnostic in most cases and liver biopsy is not needed for diagnosis.[3]

AMA are the serologic hallmark of PBC, with 98% specificity for the disease.[27] AMA targets a family of enzymes, including the pyruvate dehydrogenase complex, which catalyze the oxidative decarboxylation of keto acid substrates.[28] AMA is positive in approximately 95% of patients with PBC.[3] AMA titers vary greatly among patients, although the AMA titer does not correlate with disease severity or rate of progression.[29] Furthermore, AMA titers should not be monitored to assess for treatment efficacy. Interestingly, for those found to have elevated circulating AMA without clinically apparent liver disease or abnormal liver enzymes, AMA can be an indicator of preclinical disease, because up to 19% will develop PBC at 5 years.[30,31] Other autoantibodies are often identified and can be helpful when AMA is negative; ANA (antinuclear antibodies) is positive in 70%, and anti-Sp100 and anti-gp201 have a high specificity for PBC.[32]

Liver biopsy is not necessary to establish a PBC diagnosis. However, biopsy is helpful in cases when AMA is negative, when the clinical picture is inconsistent with PBC (ie, a young male patient), when coexisting liver conditions are suspected (ie, nonalcoholic steatohepatitis, drug injury), or when overlap syndromes (ie, with autoimmune hepatitis) are being considered. Further, biopsy can provide useful information with regard to staging and prognosis.[33] Biopsy findings include portal inflammation and asymmetric granulomatous destruction of bile ducts within portal triads with formation of granulomas. The pathognomonic florid duct lesion, an intense inflammatory infiltrate centered around intralobular bile ducts, is uncommon.[33] Histologic lesions are classically divided into 4 stages according to the degree of fibrosis, portal inflammation, and/or destruction of bile ducts (**Table 1**).[3] Although liver biopsy remains the gold standard for assessment of hepatic fibrosis, the invasive nature and potential for sampling error limits the usefulness of liver biopsy. Transient elastography has been identified as an accurate modality for identifying PBC cases associated with advanced fibrosis, and will likely be useful in longitudinal monitoring for progressive disease in patients with PBC.[34]

TREATMENT

The main goals of therapy in PBC are to halt or reverse bile duct injury, slow disease progression, improve liver function tests, and prevent the long-term consequences of

Table 1 Four histologic stages of PBC	
Stage	**Description**
1	Portal inflammation with or without florid bile duct lesions
2	Extension of inflammation to periportal areas (interface hepatitis)
3	Septal fibrosis or inflammatory bridging
4	Cirrhosis with existence of regenerative nodules
Nodular regenerative hyperplasia	Noncirrhotic complication of PBC associated with portal hypertension

Abbreviation: PBC, primary biliary cholangitis.

chronic cholestasis such as pruritus, fatigue, osteoporosis, and fat-soluble vitamin deficiencies.[35] Since the introduction and widespread use of UDCA, the clinical presentation as well as the progression of natural disease history of patients with PBC has improved significantly over the past 2 decades.[7,17] However, about one-third of patients with PBC show suboptimal biochemical responses to UDCA and remain at risk for continued progression of disease to more advanced disease, including cirrhosis.[18,36,37]

Ursodeoxycholic Acid

UDCA was the only drug approved by the US Food and Drug Administration for the treatment of PBC until the approval of obeticholic acid (OCA) in 2016.[38] UDCA is a bile acid present in human bile at a concentration of approximately 3%. Chronic cholestasis results in intrahepatic and systemic accumulation of cytotoxic bile acids that initially promote hepatocyte proliferation, but eventually leads to hepatocellular injury, apoptosis, fibrosis, and cirrhosis. UDCA has multiple mechanisms of action in cholestatic conditions including protection of cholangiocytes and periportal hepatocytes from the cytotoxic effects of hydrophobic bile acids, stimulation of hepatocellular and ductular secretion of bile acids, and hepatocyte protection against bile acid–induced apoptosis. UDCA also has additional antiinflammatory and immunomodulatory effects.[39]

The administration of UDCA increases the bile acid saturation in bile resulting in increased bile acid clearance from blood and reduced cholestatic symptoms, specifically pruritus. These effects of UDCA occur with optimal dose of 13 to 15 mg/kg/d and have been proposed to have choleretic and antiinflammatory effects.[40,41] Angulo and colleagues[41] conducted a randomized controlled trial comparing the effects of 3 doses of UDCA in the treatment of PBC. The authors concluded that a daily dose of 13 to 15 mg/kg is superior to either a lower dose or higher dose in improvement of liver biochemistries. The studies showing improvement in survival and delay the requirement of liver transplantation have used a dose of 13 to 15 mg/kg/d.

UDCA can be used for patients with abnormal liver biochemistries irrespective of histologic stage of disease.[3] Patients in the early stage of disease respond more favorably to UDCA, but multiple studies have also shown improvement in survival and avoidance of liver transplantation with use of UDCA in patients with advanced stage of disease. Poupon and colleagues[42] conducted a metaanalysis of French, Canadian, and Mayo Clinical trials and demonstrated that time to liver transplantation was significantly improved in UDCA treated patients with moderate to severe disease (serum bilirubin level of ≥ 1.4 mg/dL, stage 3 and 4 histologic abnormalities). The administration of UDCA in patients with PBC decreases the risk of hepatoma as demonstrated in multiple studies.[43,44] Kuiper and colleagues[43] demonstrated that UDCA treated patients with PBC have 3-fold decrease in the risk of hepatoma as compared with untreated patients. However, patients who show suboptimal biochemical response after 1 year of treatment with UDCA still have a significant risk for hepatoma.

Multiple studies have proposed various criteria for improvement in liver biochemistries as predictors of treatment success after treatment with UDCA. Six criteria are used more often and are summarized in **Table 2**.[7,24,26,45] These vary from 6 months after starting treatment with UDCA (Mayo Clinic criteria[24]) to 2 years (Toronto Criteria[46,47]). The other biochemical response criteria (Barcelona,[17] Paris 1,[36] Paris II,[48] and Rotterdam[37]) examine treatment response to UDCA after 1 year. Angulo and colleagues[24] showed that a Mayo risk score of less than 4.5 and/or serum ALP of less than 2 times the upper limit of normal after 6 months of UDCA treatment are predictive of a favorable response to treatment over a 2-year period (Mayo Clinic

Table 2
Biochemical response criteria

Criterion	Definition of Biochemical Response
Mayo[24]	ALP <2× ULN
Barcelona[17]	ALP decrease >40% from baseline or to normal after 1 y of UDCA.
Paris-1[36]	ALP ≤3× ULN, AST ≤2× ULN and normal bilirubin after 1 y of UDCA.
Paris-2[48]	ALP and AST ≤1.5× ULN with normal bilirubin after 1 y of UDCA.
Toronto[47]	ALP ≤1.67× ULN
Rotterdam[37]	ALP < 3× ULN, AST <2× ULN and bilirubin ≤1 mg/dL

Abbreviations: ALP, alkaline phosphatase; AST, aspartate aminotransferase; UDCA, ursodeoxycholic acid; ULN, upper limit of normal.

Criteria).[24] According to the Barcelona criteria,[17] a decrease in serum ALP of more than 40% in baseline value or a normal level after 1 year of UDCA treatment serve as a good marker of long-term prognosis. Corpechot and colleagues[36] assessed the efficiency of combinations of serum bilirubin, ALP, and AST threshold values to predict outcome after 1 year of treatment in 292 patients with PBC (Paris 1 criteria). The authors showed that patients showing ALP of less than 3 times the upper limit of normal, AST less than 2 times the upper limit of normal, and bilirubin of 1 mg/dL or greater after 1 year of UDCA had a 90% rate of transplant-free survival at 10 years as compared with 51% for those who did not (P<.001). Large cohorts from France and the United Kingdom showed that reduction of ALP to less than 1.5 times the ULN and a normal total bilirubin after 1 year of treatment with UDCA (Paris II criteria) is associated with excellent long-term survival and identified patients at low risk for disease progression.[45,48] As per the Toronto criteria,[46,47] a decrease in the serum ALP to less than 1.67 times the upper limit of normal and normalization of bilirubin after 2 year of treatment is associated with excellent long-term liver transplant-free survival.

UDCA is usually well-tolerated at the recommended dose and has minimal side effects. The most frequent adverse events reports in clinical trials are diarrhea that occurs in about 2% to 9% of cases and weight gain. Other commonly reported adverse outcomes are mild headache, right upper quadrant pain, and thinning of the hair. However, these side effects are rarely lead to discontinuation of therapy.[3,7]

In summary, the biochemical response to UDCA after 1 year of treatment is considered a strong predictor of long-term clinical outcomes. According to different biochemical response criteria in UDCA-treated patients, the inadequate response rates vary between 24% and 79%, so an approximately 40% rate of inadequate response is considered an appropriate estimation.[49] In general, a significantly large group of the patient population remains at risk for continued progression to advanced disease including cirrhosis and are in need for additional therapies.

Farnesoid X Receptor Agonists and Obeticholic Acid

OCA is a selective farnesoid X receptor (FXR) agonist derived from the primary human bile acid chenodeoxycholic acid that has been modified chemically to make it 100 times more potent than chenodeoxycholic acid.[50] The FXR nuclear receptor is expressed in the liver, intestine, adrenal glands, and kidneys. In the liver, FXR activation limits the entry of bile acids by repressing the sodium taurocholate cotransporter polypeptide, reduces the conversion of cholesterol to bile acids by down regulating cytochrome P450 7A1 (CYP7A1) and CYP8B1, the primary enzymes involved in the synthesis of bile acids and increases the expression of bilirubin exporter pumps. In the ileum, OCA decreases bile acids reabsorption by downregulating the apical sodium bile acid transporter and increasing the expression of fibroblast growth factor 19, which also decreases the bile acid production in the liver through inhibition of CYP7A1. Therefore, by activating the FXR, OCA reduces the production of bile in the liver, increases bile flow in cholestatic conditions, and thus protects hepatocytes from accumulation of cytotoxic bile acids.[51,52] OCA has shown improvement in the biochemical markers of the liver function in multiple clinical trials.[53-55]

The POISE study (PBC OCA International Study of Efficacy) was the basis for the US Food and Drug Administration's approval of OCA in the treatment of patients with PBC with inadequate response to UDCA.[55] POISE was an international, multicenter, randomized, double-blind, placebo-controlled, clinical trial that studied the safety and efficacy of OCA in patients with PBC with an incomplete response to or unable to tolerate UDCA. An inadequate response to UDCA was defined as ALP of 1.67 times the upper limit of normal or greater and/or total bilirubin of greater than the upper limit of normal but less than 2 times the upper limit of normal. Most of the participants had been on UDCA for at least 12 months and were on a stable dose for at least 3 months before enrollment. The primary endpoint was a composite of ALP level of less than 1.67 times the upper limit of normal, with a reduction of at least 15% from baseline, and a normal total bilirubin level after 12 months of therapy. Two hundred seventeen subjects were randomized to receive either placebo, 10 mg of OCA, or 5 mg of OCA titrated to 10 mg of OCA based on the basis of the side effects and biochemical response at 6 months. The composite primary endpoint was met in an intention-to-treat analysis with rates of 10% in the placebo group compared with 47% in the 10 mg OCA group and 46% in the dose-titrated 5- to 10-mg OCA group. The mean decrease in ALP from baseline was 39% in the 10-mg OCA dose group, 33% in the 5- to 10-mg titrated dose OCA group versus 5% in the placebo group.

In addition to the improvement in serum level of ALP, patients treated with a 5-mg and a 5- to 10-mg titrated dose had a greater decrease in total bilirubin compared with placebo (−0.02 and −0.05, respectively, vs 0.12). Moreover, both the OCA intervention groups met predefined secondary endpoints including significant improvement of serum AST, serum alanine aminotransferase, serum gamma glutamyl transferase, and markers of inflammation.[55]

Pruritus related to OCA was the main adverse event in the POISE trial. The incidence rates of pruritus were 38%, 56%, and 68% in the placebo, 5- to 10-mg, and 10-mg groups, respectively. The severity of pruritus was less in the titration group (<1% discontinued the trial owing to pruritus) as compared with the 10 mg OCA group (10% discontinued the trial owing to pruritus). Overall, fewer than 6% of OCA-treated patients discontinued the trial owing to pruritus.[55]

OCA has also been associated with an increase in low-density lipoprotein cholesterol and decrease in high-density lipoprotein cholesterol and triglycerides, although it is unclear whether these changes are significant clinically.[53,55]

Fibrates

Fibrates (bezafibrate and fenofibrate) may be useful for patients who had inadequate response to UDCA. Fibrates exhibit antiinflammatory and choleretic effects via activation of peroxisome proliferator activated receptor-alpha. These agents also protect the hepatobiliary system by restoring the ratio of phospholipid and bile salts to a harmless level. Multiple studies have shown improvement in liver biochemistries in patients with PBC treated with fibrates. However, improvement in survival is yet to be demonstrated.[56,57] A large randomized, double-blind, placebo-controlled trial of bezafibrate and UDCA treatment in patients with PBC with incomplete biochemical response to UCDA is currently underway (NCT01654731).

Budesonide

Budesonide is a glucocorticoid receptor (pregnane X receptor) agonist. It has very low systemic toxicity as compared with other steroids owing to first-pass metabolism in the liver. Clinical trials have shown that the combination of budesonide and UDCA improves liver biochemistries and liver histology in patients with stage 1 to stage 3 fibrosis. However, other studies showed only marginal improvement in ALP level with budesonide and also have increased side effects. Budesonide is associated with an increased risk of hepatic decompensation and portal vein thrombosis, especially when used in patients with advanced fibrosis and cirrhosis.[58,59]

Immunologic and Molecular Therapies

Owing to the immunologic nature of PBC, various immunosuppressants as well as immunomodulators have been investigated. The data on safety and efficacy of these therapies in PBC are currently lacking. Novel immunologic treatments such as anti–interleukin-12, anti-CD80, anti-CD20 (rituximab), mesenchymal stem cells, and cytotoxic T-lymphocyte antigen 4 (abatacept) are currently under investigation for the treatment of PBC.[60–62]

ANTIMITOCHONDRIAL ANTIBODY-NEGATIVE PRIMARY BILIARY CHOLANGITIS

The 5% to 10% of patients with PBC with AMA-negative disease have a similar clinical presentation, natural history, response to UDCA, and appearance on liver biopsy as AMA-positive patients.[63,64] The pathogenesis is similar, and nearly all of these patients have positive antinuclear (in particular anti-gp210 and anti-Sp100) and/or anti–smooth muscle antibodies. IgM levels tend to be lower in AMA-negative patients. Liver biopsy with features typical of bile duct destruction and/or granulomas as seen in AMA-positive PBC is necessary for diagnosis.

PRIMARY BILIARY CHOLANGITIS–ASSOCIATED SYMPTOMS AND CONDITIONS

Fatigue

Fatigue affects 4 of 5 patients with PBC and can be mild or debilitating, affecting quality of life and impacting survival. Fatigue is often intermittent and generally unrelated to disease activity or stage.[65] Although the cause is not well-understood and likely multifactorial, it seems that chronic cholestasis affects neuropsychiatric processes leading to autonomic dysfunction, sleep disturbance, and impaired concentration and memory.[7] UDCA therapy does not improve either the frequency or severity of fatigue. Modafinil, a stimulant used in narcolepsy, has been effective in small observational studies, although it has not been evaluated in randomized trials.[66,67] Other contributors to fatigue should be identified and managed, and lifestyle modifications are recommended to accommodate fatigue.

Pruritus

Pruritus is very common in PBC, affecting 20% to 70% of patients, with varying degrees of severity. Similar to fatigue, pruritus can wax and wane throughout the course of disease and is not closely related to PBC activity or stage. Early-onset pruritus, however, is associated with a more aggressive disease course with worse prognosis.[68] The pruritus of cholestasis is characterized as a deep, intense itching leading to scratching, although not relieved by scratching, and is often associated with impaired sleep and depression.[69] Cholestyramine is an anion exchange resin that lowers serum bile acids by preventing their reuptake through enterohepatic circulation. Rifampicin is recommended as a second-line therapy, although this agent requires monitoring for hepatotoxicity, renal impairment, and anemia. Opiate antagonists including naloxone and naltrexone inhibit the direct pruritogenic effect of opioids and may improve cholestasis, but use is limited by withdrawal symptoms. Sertraline, a selective serotonin reuptake inhibitor, should be considered if concomitant depression is present.[3,70]

Associated Conditions

PBC has a variety of presentations, from clinically silent with little if any liver damage, to a highly symptomatic condition associated with cirrhosis, portal hypertension, and extrahepatic manifestations, including autoimmune disease, hyperlipidemia, metabolic bone disease, and vitamin deficiencies.

Autoimmune Disease

PBC shares parallel genetic risk factors with other autoimmune conditions; more than one-half of patients with PBC have a concomitant autoimmune disease.[71] Antinuclear antibodies and anti–smooth muscle antibodies are also found in nearly one-half of patients with PBC.[4] The strongest association is with Sjögren syndrome, a chronic autoimmune disorder of the exocrine glands, with a reported prevalence of up to 40% among patients with PBC.[72,73] The most common symptoms of Sjögren syndrome are dry eyes and mouth, known as Sicca complex, although these symptoms are common in PBC in the absence of Sjögren syndrome. Both Sjögren syndrome and sicca symptoms are likely mediated by autoimmune destruction of epithelial targets shared by exocrine glands and biliary tract. Associated symptoms should be addressed and managed, often with supportive therapy alone. Autoimmune thyroid disease, CREST syndrome (calcinosis, Raynaud phenomenon, esophageal dysmotility, sclerodactyly, and telangiectasia), rheumatoid arthritis, and Raynaud syndrome are other common concomitant conditions, particularly in women.[7]

Hyperlipidemia

Elevated serum lipids are seen almost universally in PBC; hyperlipidemia affects 75% to 95% of patients.[74] The mechanism of hyperlipidemia in PBC is unique and related to cholestasis. High-density lipoprotein cholesterol is disproportionately increased and other lipoprotein particles accumulate to increase total cholesterol. The hyperlipidemia associated with PBC is not associated with increased atherosclerotic risk or cardiovascular disease.[75,76] Lipid-lowering agents, namely statins, can be safely used if indicated for other reasons such as presence of the metabolic syndrome or a family history of coronary artery disease.[77] UDCA and OCA are associated with modest reductions in lipid levels via reduction of cholestasis.[53,78] Xanthomas, deposits of cholesterol in the skin, and xanthelasmas, cholesterol deposits in the medial eyelids, are rare, and develop when serum cholesterol is markedly elevated over time.

Metabolic Bone Disease

The majority of patients with PBC have osteopenia, and approximately one-third have osteoporosis. The relative risk of osteoporosis in PBC as compared with age- and sex-matched controls is 4.4.[79] The cause of osteopenic bone disease is multifactorial and related to some degree to chronic cholestasis with altered bone resorption and formation, in addition to higher rates in PBC of known risk factors including female sex, low body mass index, advanced age, and advanced liver disease.[80,81] Vitamin D

Box 1
Follow-up of PBC

Monitor liver enzymes every 3 to 6 months

Annual TSH, vitamin D, and lipid panel

Bone mineral density scan every 2 to 4 years

Monitor and manage symptoms: fatigue, pruritus, sicca syndrome

Upper endoscopy for varices screen once cirrhosis diagnosed or Mayo risk score of greater than 4.1 or platelets less than 140,000/mm^3

PBC with cirrhosis
   Monitoring of liver function
   Screening and management of varices
   Ultrasound examination and alpha fetoprotein every 6 months

Abbreviations: PBC, primary biliary cholangitis; TSH, thyroid-stimulating hormone.

---

deficiency occurs in 13% to 33% of patients with PBC, but is often seen in more severe liver disease and does not fully explain the osteopenia of PBC.[82] Patients with PBC should have a bone mineral density test (ie, dual-energy x-ray absorptiometry) at diagnosis and for surveillance every 2 to 4 years, and be counseled on lifestyle interventions to promote bone health (ie, smoking cessation, alcohol moderation, weight bearing exercises). Calcium and vitamin D should be supplemented for patients with osteopenia, and bisphosphonate therapy should be considered for those with osteoporosis, in the absence of esophageal varices.[81]

Vitamin Deficiencies

Patients with chronic cholestasis have increased risk of lipid malabsorption and therefore malabsorption of the fat-soluble vitamins (vitamins A, D, E, and K). Vitamin A deficiency can affect night vision, vitamin D deficiency affects bone health, vitamin E deficiency can lead to peripheral neuropathy and immune dysfunction, and vitamin K deficiency can affect clotting factors.[83] The recommendation is to test vitamin A, D, and K levels annually.[3] Follow-up on patients with PBC are summarized in **Box 1**.

SUMMARY

PBC is an increasingly recognized chronic autoimmune liver disease characterized by progressive destruction of intrahepatic bile ducts, cholestasis, portal inflammation, and in some cases, cirrhosis and portal hypertension. PBC is likely in patients with elevated ALP and AMA, and is classically seen in middle-aged women who present without symptoms or with fatigue and itching. The pathogenesis is incompletely understood, but involves both genetic susceptibility and environmental triggers. The prognosis of PBC has improved significantly with disease recognition and diagnosis at earlier stages, and the widespread use of UDCA as a treatment. OCA has been approved recently as a second-line therapy. There are a number of complications of chronic cholestasis and conditions associated with PBC that should be recognized and appropriately managed. Although patients with early stage disease have a normal life expectancy, fatigue and pruritus, which are not correlated with stage of disease and are not relieved by UDCA or OCA therapy, can be debilitating and negatively impact quality of life. An improved understanding of the pathogenesis and molecular pathways that underlie PBC may lead to advent of targeted effective therapy to halt disease progression and manage associated symptoms.

REFERENCES

1. Boonstra K, Beuers U, Ponsioen CY. Epidemiology of primary sclerosing cholangitis and primary biliary cirrhosis: a systematic review. J Hepatol 2012;56(5): 1181–8.
2. Boonstra K, Kunst AE, Stadhouders PH, et al. Rising incidence and prevalence of primary biliary cirrhosis: a large population-based study. Liver Int 2014;34(6): e31–8.
3. Lindor KD, Gershwin ME, Poupon R, et al. Primary biliary cirrhosis. Hepatology 2009;50(1):291–308.
4. Kaplan MM, Gershwin ME. Primary biliary cirrhosis. N Engl J Med 2005;353(12): 1261–73.
5. Jones DE. Pathogenesis of primary biliary cirrhosis. J Hepatol 2003;39(4): 639–48.
6. Selmi C, Bowlus CL, Gershwin ME, et al. Primary biliary cirrhosis. Lancet 2011; 377(9777):1600–9.
7. Carey EJ, Ali AH, Lindor KD. Primary biliary cirrhosis. Lancet 2015;386(10003): 1565–75.
8. McNally RJ, James PW, Ducker S, et al. No rise in incidence but geographical heterogeneity in the occurrence of primary biliary cirrhosis in North East England. Am J Epidemiol 2014;179(4):492–8.
9. Bach N, Schaffner F. Familial primary biliary cirrhosis. J Hepatol 1994;20(6): 698–701.
10. Kaplan MM, Bianchi DW. Primary biliary cirrhosis: for want of an X chromosome? Lancet 2004;363(9408):505–6.
11. Prince M, Chetwynd A, Newman W, et al. Survival and symptom progression in a geographically based cohort of patients with primary biliary cirrhosis: follow-up for up to 28 years. Gastroenterology 2002;123(4):1044–51.
12. Locke GR 3rd, Therneau TM, Ludwig J, et al. Time course of histological progression in primary biliary cirrhosis. Hepatology 1996;23(1):52–6.
13. Lindor KD, Jorgensen RA, Therneau TM, et al. Ursodeoxycholic acid delays the onset of esophageal varices in primary biliary cirrhosis. Mayo Clin Proc 1997; 72(12):1137–40.
14. Poupon RE, Lindor KD, Pares A, et al. Combined analysis of the effect of treatment with ursodeoxycholic acid on histologic progression in primary biliary cirrhosis. J Hepatol 2003;39(1):12–6.
15. Imam MH, Lindor KD. The natural history of primary biliary cirrhosis. Semin Liver Dis 2014;34(3):329–33.
16. Lammers WJ, van Buuren HR, Hirschfield GM, et al. Levels of alkaline phosphatase and bilirubin are surrogate end points of outcomes of patients with primary biliary cirrhosis: an international follow-up study. Gastroenterology 2014;147(6): 1338–49.e5 [quiz: e1315].
17. Pares A, Caballeria L, Rodes J. Excellent long-term survival in patients with primary biliary cirrhosis and biochemical response to ursodeoxycholic acid. Gastroenterology 2006;130(3):715–20.
18. Carbone M, Mells GF, Pells G, et al. Sex and age are determinants of the clinical phenotype of primary biliary cirrhosis and response to ursodeoxycholic acid. Gastroenterology 2013;144(3):560–9.e7 [quiz: e513–64].

19. Christensen E, Altman DG, Neuberger J, et al. Updating prognosis in primary biliary cirrhosis using a time-dependent Cox regression model. PBC1 and PBC2 trial groups. Gastroenterology 1993;105(6):1865–76.

20. Christensen E, Neuberger J, Crowe J, et al. Beneficial effect of azathioprine and prediction of prognosis in primary biliary cirrhosis. Final results of an international trial. Gastroenterology 1985;89(5):1084–91.

21. Dickson ER, Grambsch PM, Fleming TR, et al. Prognosis in primary biliary cirrhosis: model for decision making. Hepatology 1989;10(1):1–7.

22. Roll J, Boyer JL, Barry D, et al. The prognostic importance of clinical and histologic features in asymptomatic and symptomatic primary biliary cirrhosis. N Engl J Med 1983;308(1):1–7.

23. van Dam GM, Verbaan BW, Therneau TM, et al. Primary biliary cirrhosis: Dutch application of the Mayo Model before and after orthotopic liver transplantation. Hepatogastroenterology 1997;44(15):732–43.

24. Angulo P, Lindor KD, Therneau TM, et al. Utilization of the Mayo risk score in patients with primary biliary cirrhosis receiving ursodeoxycholic acid. Liver 1999; 19(2):115–21.

25. Corpechot C, Carrat F, Bahr A, et al. The effect of ursodeoxycholic acid therapy on the natural course of primary biliary cirrhosis. Gastroenterology 2005;128(2): 297–303.

26. Lammers WJ, Hirschfield GM, Corpechot C, et al. Development and validation of a scoring system to predict outcomes of patients with primary biliary cirrhosis receiving ursodeoxycholic acid therapy. Gastroenterology 2015;149(7): 1804–12.e4.

27. Van de Water J, Cooper A, Surh CD, et al. Detection of autoantibodies to recombinant mitochondrial proteins in patients with primary biliary cirrhosis. N Engl J Med 1989;320(21):1377–80.

28. Moteki S, Leung PS, Dickson ER, et al. Epitope mapping and reactivity of autoantibodies to the E2 component of 2-oxoglutarate dehydrogenase complex in primary biliary cirrhosis using recombinant 2-oxoglutarate dehydrogenase complex. Hepatology 1996;23(3):436–44.

29. Van Norstrand MD, Malinchoc M, Lindor KD, et al. Quantitative measurement of autoantibodies to recombinant mitochondrial antigens in patients with primary biliary cirrhosis: relationship of levels of autoantibodies to disease progression. Hepatology 1997;25(1):6–11.

30. Dahlqvist G, Corpechot C. Are antimitochondrial antibodies the invariable hallmark of primary biliary cirrhosis? Presse Med 2014;43(12 Pt 1):1311–3 [in French].

31. Mattalia A, Quaranta S, Leung PS, et al. Characterization of antimitochondrial antibodies in health adults. Hepatology 1998;27(3):656–61.

32. Nakamura M, Kondo H, Mori T, et al. Anti-gp210 and anti-centromere antibodies are different risk factors for the progression of primary biliary cirrhosis. Hepatology 2007;45(1):118–27.

33. Zein CO, Angulo P, Lindor KD. When is liver biopsy needed in the diagnosis of primary biliary cirrhosis? Clin Gastroenterol Hepatol 2003;1(2):89–95.

34. Corpechot C, Carrat F, Poujol-Robert A, et al. Noninvasive elastography-based assessment of liver fibrosis progression and prognosis in primary biliary cirrhosis. Hepatology 2012;56(1):198–208.

35. Czul F, Peyton A, Levy C. Primary biliary cirrhosis: therapeutic advances. Clin Liver Dis 2013;17(2):229–42.

36. Corpechot C, Abenavoli L, Rabahi N, et al. Biochemical response to ursodeoxycholic acid and long-term prognosis in primary biliary cirrhosis. Hepatology 2008; 48(3):871–7.

37. Kuiper EM, Hansen BE, de Vries RA, et al. Improved prognosis of patients with primary biliary cirrhosis that have a biochemical response to ursodeoxycholic acid. Gastroenterology 2009;136(4):1281–7.

38. Bowlus CL. Obeticholic acid for the treatment of primary biliary cholangitis in adult patients: clinical utility and patient selection. Hepat Med 2016;8:89–95.

39. Poupon R. Ursodeoxycholic acid and bile-acid mimetics as therapeutic agents for cholestatic liver diseases: an overview of their mechanisms of action. Clin Res Hepatol Gastroenterol 2012;36(Suppl 1):S3–12.

40. Angulo P, Batts KP, Therneau TM, et al. Long-term ursodeoxycholic acid delays histological progression in primary biliary cirrhosis. Hepatology 1999;29(3): 644–7.

41. Angulo P, Dickson ER, Therneau TM, et al. Comparison of three doses of ursodeoxycholic acid in the treatment of primary biliary cirrhosis: a randomized trial. J Hepatol 1999;30(5):830–5.

42. Poupon RE, Lindor KD, Cauch-Dudek K, et al. Combined analysis of randomized controlled trials of ursodeoxycholic acid in primary biliary cirrhosis. Gastroenterology 1997;113(3):884–90.

43. Kuiper EM, Hansen BE, Adang RP, et al. Relatively high risk for hepatocellular carcinoma in patients with primary biliary cirrhosis not responding to ursodeoxycholic acid. Eur J Gastroenterol Hepatol 2010;22(12):1495–502.

44. Zhang XX, Wang LF, Jin L, et al. Primary biliary cirrhosis-associated hepatocellular carcinoma in Chinese patients: incidence and risk factors. World J Gastroenterol 2015;21(12):3554–63.

45. Papastergiou V, Tsochatzis EA, Rodriguez-Peralvarez M, et al. Biochemical criteria at 1 year are not robust indicators of response to ursodeoxycholic acid in early primary biliary cirrhosis: results from a 29-year cohort study. Aliment Pharmacol Ther 2013;38(11–12):1354–64.

46. Kumagi T, Guindi M, Fischer SE, et al. Baseline ductopenia and treatment response predict long-term histological progression in primary biliary cirrhosis. Am J Gastroenterol 2010;105(10):2186–94.

47. Lammert C, Juran BD, Schlicht E, et al. Biochemical response to ursodeoxycholic acid predicts survival in a North American cohort of primary biliary cirrhosis patients. J Gastroenterol 2014;49(10):1414–20.

48. Corpechot C, Chazouilleres O, Poupon R. Early primary biliary cirrhosis: biochemical response to treatment and prediction of long-term outcome. J Hepatol 2011;55(6):1361–7.

49. van Buuren HR, Lammers WJ, Harms MH, et al. Surrogate endpoints for optimal therapeutic response to UDCA in primary biliary cholangitis. Dig Dis 2015; 33(Suppl 2):118–24.

50. Pellicciari R, Fiorucci S, Camaioni E, et al. 6alpha-ethyl-chenodeoxycholic acid (6-ECDCA), a potent and selective FXR agonist endowed with anticholestatic activity. J Med Chem 2002;45(17):3569–72.

51. Flores A, Mayo MJ. Primary biliary cirrhosis in 2014. Curr Opin Gastroenterol 2014;30(3):245–52.

52. Lindor KD. Farnesoid X receptor agonists for primary biliary cirrhosis. Curr Opin Gastroenterol 2011;27(3):285–8.

53. Hirschfield GM, Mason A, Luketic V, et al. Efficacy of obeticholic acid in patients with primary biliary cirrhosis and inadequate response to ursodeoxycholic acid. Gastroenterology 2015;148(4):751–61.e8.

54. Kowdley KV, Jones DE, Luketic V. The OCA PBC Study Group, an international study evaluating the farnesoid X receptor agonist obeticholic acid as monotherapy in PBC. J Hepatol 2012;54:S13.

55. Nevens F, Andreone P, Mazzella G, et al. A placebo-controlled trial of obeticholic acid in primary biliary cholangitis. N Engl J Med 2016;375(7):631–43.

56. Hazzan R, Tur-Kaspa R. Bezafibrate treatment of primary biliary cirrhosis following incomplete response to ursodeoxycholic acid. J Clin Gastroenterol 2010;44(5):371–3.

57. Honda A, Ikegami T, Nakamuta M, et al. Anticholestatic effects of bezafibrate in patients with primary biliary cirrhosis treated with ursodeoxycholic acid. Hepatology 2013;57(5):1931–41.

58. Leuschner M, Maier KP, Schlichting J, et al. Oral budesonide and ursodeoxycholic acid for treatment of primary biliary cirrhosis: results of a prospective double-blind trial. Gastroenterology 1999;117(4):918–25.

59. Rautiainen H, Karkkainen P, Karvonen AL, et al. Budesonide combined with UDCA to improve liver histology in primary biliary cirrhosis: a three-year randomized trial. Hepatology 2005;41(4):747–52.

60. Beuers U, Gershwin ME. Unmet challenges in immune-mediated hepatobiliary diseases. Clin Rev Allergy Immunol 2015;48(2–3):127–31.

61. Invernizzi P, Gershwin ME. New therapeutics in primary biliary cirrhosis: will there ever be light? Liver Int 2014;34(2):167–70.

62. Tsuda M, Moritoki Y, Lian ZX, et al. Biochemical and immunologic effects of rituximab in patients with primary biliary cirrhosis and an incomplete response to ursodeoxycholic acid. Hepatology 2012;55(2):512–21.

63. Lacerda MA, Ludwig J, Dickson ER, et al. Antimitochondrial antibody-negative primary biliary cirrhosis. Am J Gastroenterol 1995;90(2):247–9.

64. Mendes F, Lindor KD. Antimitochondrial antibody-negative primary biliary cirrhosis. Gastroenterol Clin North Am 2008;37(2):479–84, viii.

65. Jopson L, Jones DE. Fatigue in primary biliary cirrhosis: prevalence, pathogenesis and management. Dig Dis 2015;33(Suppl 2):109–14.

66. Jones DE, Newton JL. An open study of modafinil for the treatment of daytime somnolence and fatigue in primary biliary cirrhosis. Aliment Pharmacol Ther 2007;25(4):471–6.

67. Ian Gan S, de Jongh M, Kaplan MM. Modafinil in the treatment of debilitating fatigue in primary biliary cirrhosis: a clinical experience. Dig Dis Sci 2009;54(10):2242–6.

68. Quarneti C, Muratori P, Lalanne C, et al. Fatigue and pruritus at onset identify a more aggressive subset of primary biliary cirrhosis. Liver Int 2015;35(2):636–41.

69. Beuers U, Kremer AE, Bolier R, et al. Pruritus in cholestasis: facts and fiction. Hepatology 2014;60(1):399–407.

70. Kremer AE, Namer B, Bolier R, et al. Pathogenesis and management of pruritus in PBC and PSC. Dig Dis 2015;33(Suppl 2):164–75.

71. Corpechot C, Chretien Y, Chazouilleres O, et al. Demographic, lifestyle, medical and familial factors associated with primary biliary cirrhosis. J Hepatol 2010;53(1):162–9.

72. Floreani A, Spinazze A, Caballeria L, et al. Extrahepatic malignancies in primary biliary cirrhosis: a comparative study at two European centers. Clin Rev Allergy Immunol 2015;48(2–3):254–62.

73. Liu B, Zhang FC, Zhang ZL, et al. Interstitial lung disease and Sjogren's syndrome in primary biliary cirrhosis: a causal or casual association? Clin Rheumatol 2008; 27(10):1299–306.
74. Sorokin A, Brown JL, Thompson PD. Primary biliary cirrhosis, hyperlipidemia, and atherosclerotic risk: a systematic review. Atherosclerosis 2007;194(2):293–9.
75. Allocca M, Crosignani A, Gritti A, et al. Hypercholesterolaemia is not associated with early atherosclerotic lesions in primary biliary cirrhosis. Gut 2006;55(12): 1795–800.
76. Longo M, Crosignani A, Battezzati PM, et al. Hyperlipidaemic state and cardio-vascular risk in primary biliary cirrhosis. Gut 2002;51(2):265–9.
77. Cash WJ, O'Neill S, O'Donnell ME, et al. Randomized controlled trial assessing the effect of simvastatin in primary biliary cirrhosis. Liver Int 2013;33(8):1166–74.
78. Balan V, Dickson ER, Jorgensen RA, et al. Effect of ursodeoxycholic acid on serum lipids of patients with primary biliary cirrhosis. Mayo Clin Proc 1994; 69(10):923–9.
79. Southerland JC, Valentine JF. Osteopenia and osteoporosis in gastrointestinal diseases: diagnosis and treatment. Curr Gastroenterol Rep 2001;3(5):399–407.
80. Guanabens N, Pares A, Ros I, et al. Severity of cholestasis and advanced histo-logical stage but not menopausal status are the major risk factors for osteoporosis in primary biliary cirrhosis. J Hepatol 2005;42(4):573–7.
81. Guanabens N, Monegal A, Cerda D, et al. Randomized trial comparing monthly ibandronate and weekly alendronate for osteoporosis in patients with primary biliary cirrhosis. Hepatology 2013;58(6):2070–8.
82. Agmon-Levin N, Kopilov R, Selmi C, et al. Vitamin D in primary biliary cirrhosis, a plausible marker of advanced disease. Immunol Res 2015;61(1–2):141–6.
83. Phillips JR, Angulo P, Petterson T, et al. Fat-soluble vitamin levels in patients with primary biliary cirrhosis. Am J Gastroenterol 2001;96(9):2745–50.

Primary Sclerosing Cholangitis
What the Gastroenterologist and Hepatologist Needs to Know

Andrea A. Gossard, APRN, CNP*, Gregory J. Gores, MD

KEYWORDS

- Biliary tract disease • Cholangiocarcinoma • Cholestasis
- Inflammatory bowel disease • Liver disease • Primary sclerosing cholangitis

KEY POINTS

- Primary sclerosing cholangitis (PSC) is an idiopathic biliary tract disease characterized by bile duct inflammation and fibrosis which may progress to cirrhosis and end-stage liver disease.
- The majority of patients with PSC are male and nearly 80% also have inflammatory bowel disease (IBD).
- Diagnostic criteria for PSC include aberrations in liver enzymes with characteristic bile duct irregularities identified by cholangiographic imaging.
- PSC is associated with an increased risk for developing cholangiocarcinoma. Surveillance with imaging and a serum carbohydrate antigen 19-9 may be performed annually.
- The risk of colorectal cancer is significantly increased for patients with PSC and IBD. Surveillance colonoscopy should be performed every 1 to 2 years.

DOES MY PATIENT HAVE PRIMARY SCLEROSING CHOLANGITIS?

Primary sclerosing cholangitis (PSC) is a chronic, idiopathic liver condition characterized by biliary tract inflammation and ultimately bile duct destruction by a fibrous, obliterative process.[1,2] The diagnosis is based on several key diagnostic criteria, including serum liver tests, typically elevated in a cholestatic profile, and classic bile duct changes noted on direct or indirect cholangiography (**Box 1**). The disease is often progressive, leading to fibrosis, cirrhosis, and end-stage liver disease.[3] The natural history of the condition is variable, however, with a subset of patients progressing relatively

Disclosures: The authors have nothing to disclose.
Division of Gastroenterology and Hepatology, Mayo Clinic, 200 1st Street Southwest, Rochester, MN 55901, USA
* Corresponding author.
E-mail address: Gossard.andrea@mayo.edu

Clin Liver Dis 21 (2017) 725–737
http://dx.doi.org/10.1016/j.cld.2017.06.004
liver.theclinics.com

> **Box 1**
> **Diagnostic criteria for primary sclerosing cholangitis**
>
> *Blood work*
> - Liver enzyme elevations in a cholestatic profile
>
> *Indirect or direct cholangiography*
> - Bile duct irregularity with segmental strictures and areas of dilation
> - Bile duct wall thickening and enhancement on magnetic resonance cholangiopancreatography
>
> *Histopathology (biopsy is not typically needed)*
> - Mixed inflammatory cell infiltrate
> - Periductal fibrosis
>
> *Other*
> - 70% to 80% will have coexistent inflammatory bowel disease
> - Male predominance

rapidly whereas others experience a more indolent course, which may span years or even decades. Oftentimes, there are no clinical symptoms at the time of presentation and blood work abnormalities are an incidental finding. Other times, the patient may present with pruritus, abdominal discomfort in the right upper quadrant, or symptoms of acute bacterial cholangitis. For some patients, the diagnosis is established as part of a comprehensive evaluation of the patient newly diagnosed with inflammatory bowel disease (IBD).

Demographics

The prevalence and incidence of PSC varies in different regions of the world.[4] The prevalence in North America and Europe ranges from 6 to 16 cases per 100,000 individuals.[5,6] The incidence ranges from 0 to 1.3 cases per 100,000 per year.[7] It is estimated that there are approximately 29,000 people with the condition in the United States.[5] The median age of patients diagnosed with PSC is 41 years of age and the disease is more common among males than females.[8] Of patients with PSC, 70% to 80% have IBD, most often chronic ulcerative colitis, whereas only 4% of patients with chronic ulcerative colitis have PSC.[9]

Biochemistries

Approximately 50% of patients with PSC have no clinical symptoms, but are diagnosed after liver enzyme elevations are detected on routine blood work.[10,11] Most often, these elevations have a cholestatic nature with elevations of the serum alkaline phosphatase more prominently than elevations of the aminotransferases. Bilirubin levels are often normal at diagnosis, but can become elevated in the setting of bile duct obstruction or with progressive liver disease. The level of serum albumin and prothrombin time are typically normal in early PSC. Autoantibody assessment is typically not helpful. Anti–neutrophil-specific antibodies are, however, detected in 80% to 88% of patients with PSC, but the clinical significance of this finding is unclear.[12,13]

Imaging

When PSC is suspected, cross-sectional imaging may be performed to evaluate for abnormalities of the liver and biliary tract. Perhaps the most useful modality is magnetic resonance cholangiopancreatography (MRCP). This imaging modality allows the radiologist to indirectly visualize the bile ducts to evaluate for fibrotic changes of the biliary tree, inflammatory strictures, or areas of bile duct dilation. Classic features of PSC include multifocal stricturing within the intrahepatic and/ or extrahepatic bile ducts with associated upstream dilation (**Fig. 1**). Most often, these changes are diffuse; however, in perhaps 20%, the changes only involve the intrahepatic ducts.[14] A cholestatic biochemical profile and MRCP showing classic diffuse biliary changes of PSC is sufficient to make a diagnosis of PSC.

Endoscopic Retrograde Cholangiopancreatography

The clinical need for diagnostic endoscopic retrograde cholangiopancreatography (ERCP) has decreased owing to the availability of MRCP. Therapeutic ERCP is appropriate if a patient with PSC develops pain, an abrupt change in serum bilirubin, acute bacterial cholangitis, and/or progressive dominant strictures on MRCP. Dominant strictures are defined as stenoses with a diameter of 1.5 mm in the common bile duct or 1 mm in the intrahepatic duct (**Fig. 2**). They develop in about 50% of patients with PSC and may lead to significant biliary obstruction.[15] For these patients, therapeutic ERCP can be performed to dilate and potentially stent biliary strictures.[9] Furthermore, biliary tissue acquisition can be achieved by brush cytology and or intraductal biopsy during ERCP and is helpful in distinguishing benign from malignant strictures.[16]

Liver Biopsy

Liver biopsy is not typically required to diagnose PSC. An exception to this is suspicion of PSC in the setting of known IBD and increased liver enzyme, but a normal cholangiogram. These patients may have a variant of PSC known as small duct PSC. This group comprises perhaps 5% of all PSC.[17] Patients with small duct PSC survive longer and have a lower cumulative risk for cholangiocarcinoma (CCA) over a 7- to 10-year period when compared with their counterparts with large duct disease.[18,19] Approximately 20% of patients diagnosed with small duct PSC will develop features of large duct disease after 7 to 10 years.[18,19]

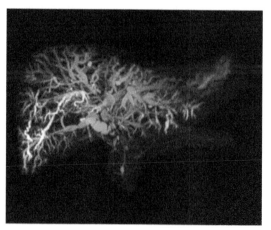

Fig. 1. Magnetic resonance cholangiopancreatography showing classic changes of primary sclerosing cholangitis.

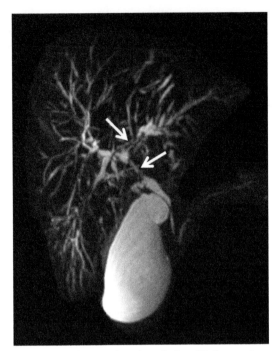

Fig. 2. Dominant strictures in primary sclerosing cholangitis (*arrows*).

Overlap syndromes in the setting of PSC do occur. Approximately 35% of children diagnosed with PSC have concurrent features of autoimmune hepatitis.[20] In the adult population, however, this occurs in only 5% of all cases.[21] If autoimmune hepatitis overlap is confirmed, appropriate treatment with corticosteroid monotherapy or a combination approach with the addition of a steroid-sparing agent is recommended. A liver biopsy is indicated to make the diagnosis of PSC with autoimmune hepatitis. This overlap syndrome is usually suspected when there is a disproportionate elevation of the serum aminotransferases. Gamma globulin can be increased in PSC as well, and does not differentiate PSC from overlap syndromes.

HOW DO I MANAGE MY PATIENT WITH PRIMARY SCLEROSING CHOLANGITIS?
Treatment Options

To date, there is no known effective therapy to treat PSC. Perhaps the most studied therapy is ursodeoxycholic acid (UDCA) given its benefit in primary biliary cholangitis.[22,23] A metaanalysis of 8 clinical trials, however, determined that UDCA did not slow the progression of PSC.[24] That said, at doses of 15 mg/kg/d, there may be a benefit. Several recent studies have suggested that patients who normalize their liver biochemistries at a moderate dose of UDCA have a better prognosis,[25,26] in particular, patients who normalize their serum alkaline phosphatase level.[25] Based on this observation, many clinicians prescribe UDCA to determine if the serum alkaline phosphatase normalizes. If it does, they continue therapy indefinitely. If there is no change in serum liver biochemistries after 6 months, the UDCA is discontinued.[27] Furthermore, some patients experience clinical improvement while on UDCA that deteriorates when treatment is discontinued.[28]

Investigational trials are underway with hopes of identifying an effective treatment. Obeticholic acid is a semisynthetic bile acid analogue that is an farnesoid X receptor agonist. Obeticholic acid is approved by the US Food and Drug Association for the treatment of primary biliary cholangitis. Studies evaluating its efficacy as treatment of PSC are underway. Immunosuppressive therapies have been tried and have not demonstrated clinical benefit for patients with PSC. As such, they do not have a role in the management of this condition.[9,29–31] There have been anecdotal reports and case series data that support use of oral vancomycin to reduce liver biochemistries and to improve clinical symptoms, particularly in the pediatric population.[32,33] Further investigation, however, is needed. In the absence of known effective therapy, patients should be encouraged to consider clinical trial participation when available.

Surveillance

Patients with PSC have an almost 400-fold increased risk of developing CCA when compared with the general population.[34] CCA occurs in 1% to 2% of patients with PSC each year with a 30-year incidence of 20%.[34–36] Regular surveillance for the development of CCA is encouraged as a part of the management strategy for patients with PSC. Of importance, the presence of advanced fibrosis is not necessary for the development of CCA, unlike hepatocellular carcinoma, which is typically found in the setting of cirrhosis. Although described, hepatocellular carcinoma in PSC is rare.[37,38]

Clinical features worrisome for CCA include weight loss, jaundice, elevations in serum carbohydrate antigen (CA) 19-9, and hyperbilirubinemia. If patients present with these symptoms, imaging should be performed to evaluate for a malignant stricture (**Fig. 3**). Dominant strictures in the setting of an elevated CA 19-9 and clinical jaundice are worrisome for CCA and direct sampling with brushings and potentially intraductal biopsy should be performed. Differentiating benign versus malignant strictures in the setting of PSC is challenging based on imaging alone.

Because CCA is difficult to diagnose, screening with imaging via ultrasound or MRI along with serum carbohydrate antigen 19-9 (CA 19–9) every 12 months is recommended.[39,40] Although the CA 19-9 alone is not sensitive nor specific enough to detect CCA, values greater than 130 U/L in the absence of bacterial cholangitis are 79% sensitive and 98% specific for CCA.[41] As such, further investigation is strongly recommended in this setting.

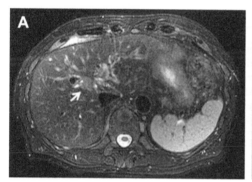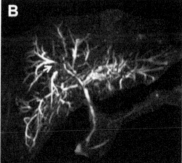

Fig. 3. Magnetic resonance imaging (A) with magnetic resonance cholangiopancreatography (B) of asymptomatic male with primary sclerosing cholangitis who was identified as having cholangiocarcinoma on surveillance imaging. Arrows designate the malignant stricture and mass.

In addition to imaging and a serum CA 19-9, ERCP can help to establish the diagnosis of malignancy. Conventional cytology has a low sensitivity (<40%) but the specificity is nearly 100%.[9] Fluorescence in situ hybridization (FISH) for identifying chromosomal aberrations, namely increased copy number variation, is an advanced cytologic technique for the diagnosis of CCA.[42,43] FISH demonstrated equal specificity but greater sensitivity when compared with cytology.[43] FISH requires a probe set applied to subpopulations of cells with chromosome amplifications to assess copy number variation termed aneusomy. In the presence of aneusomy, the additional copies of chromosomal loci are detected by the FISH probes. Results are assigned to 1 of 3 categories: negative, trisomy or tetrasomy (3 or 4 amplifications of a single locus), or polysomy (amplification of $\geq$2 loci). Among patients with PSC and a dominant stricture, the presence of polysomy identified those who eventually developed CCA with 88% specificity.[44]

Patients with PSC are also at an increased risk for the development of gallbladder malignancy. In fact, approximately 60% of gallbladder lesions in this setting are indeed adenocarcinomas.[45,46] In addition to CCA surveillance, patients with PSC should be monitored for the development of gallbladder cancer. Although small gallbladder polyps may be followed, those that exceed 8 mm in size should be removed with cholecystectomy.[47]

WHAT IS RECOMMENDED FOR MY PATIENT WITH PRIMARY SCLEROSING CHOLANGITIS AND INFLAMMATORY BOWEL DISEASE?
Colorectal Cancer Screening

The majority of patients with PSC and IBD are diagnosed with IBD before the PSC diagnosis is known. For many patients with both conditions, the IBD may be relatively quiescent. For those without a diagnosis of IBD at the time of PSC diagnosis, baseline colonoscopy to screen for this condition is recommended. In the event there is no evidence of IBD, follow-up colonoscopy should be performed in 5 years to evaluate for the development of the disease, sooner if symptoms develop.

IBD in the setting of PSC seems to be unique in that there is a predilection to right-sided colonic involvement, backwash ileitis, and rectal sparing when compared with patients with IBD but no PSC. The risk of colorectal cancer is 4- to 5-fold higher in the setting of PSC and IBD versus IBD alone.[48] When compared with the general population, the risk of colorectal cancer is 10-fold higher.[49] As such, colonoscopy with surveillance biopsies is recommended for these patients every 1 to 2 years.

Inflammatory Bowel Disease Drugs and Primary Sclerosing Cholangitis

The vast majority of therapies prescribed for IBD including aminosalicylates, 6-mercaptopurine, and corticosteroids are considered safe in the setting of PSC (**Box 2**). That said, monitoring serum liver tests after initiation of new treatments is in order to evaluate for drug-induced liver injury. There has been a fair amount of interest in novel pharmacologic therapies including immunomodulators and biologics as potential treatment for both IBD and PSC, but further study is needed with regard to potential benefit for patients with PSC.

WHAT ARE THE COMPLICATIONS OF PRIMARY SCLEROSING CHOLANGITIS AND HOW DO I MANAGE THEM?
Biliary Tract Obstruction

Patients with PSC are at risk for biliary strictures and associated obstructive symptoms (ie, pruritus, jaundice, acute bacterial cholangitis). These clinical symptoms

---

Box 2
Treatments for inflammatory bowel disease considered safe in primary sclerosing cholangitis

Antiinflammatory

Aminosalicylates

Corticosteroids

Immunosuppressants

Azathioprine

6-Mercaptopurine

Tumor necrosis factor-alpha inhibitors ("biologics")

Methotrexate

Antibiotics

Metronidazole

Ciprofloxacin

Antidiarrheals

Psyllium

Methylcellulose

Loperamide

---

and laboratory observations should warrant further investigation. Biliary strictures may occur in the intrahepatic or extrahepatic biliary tree, and can be present at the time of diagnosis or may develop years later. Although patients with mild stricturing are likely to be asymptomatic, those with dominant strictures oftentimes will have symptoms such as right upper quadrant pain, jaundice, and pruritus. Acholic stools, dark urine and fevers may also develop. Such symptoms and findings warrant either indirect (MRCP) or direct cholangiography (ERCP).

Endoscopic therapy should be considered if imaging suggests a biliary stricture in the large intrahepatic or the extrahepatic ducts on MRCP.[50,51] Although the exact prevalence of dominant strictures is unknown, approximately 50% of patients with PSC will eventually develop such strictures.[15] Those that are symptomatic are less common, occurring in 10% to 30% of patients with PSC.[15,52] Balloon dilation alone or with stent placement can improve obstructive symptoms; however, stenting should be reserved for situations where dilation alone is unable to maintain luminal patentcy.[52] The duration of stenting is variable, but may span up to 6 to 8 weeks. Prolonged stenting may increase the risk of complications and should be avoided.[53] However, some patients will require repeat stenting over a period of weeks to months to adequately treat severe strictures.

Percutaneous approaches to access the biliary tree may be considered for patients with altered anatomy, such as in the setting of previous gastric bypass or owing to failed endoscopic attempts. This process should be reserved as a second-line approach however, owing to the increased risks associated with the procedure. These risks include complications such as hemobilia, hepatic artery injury, and cholangitis.[54–56] The percutaneous approach is more invasive than an ERCP and stenting via this approach is more problematic for the patient (management of the external biliary tube).

Cholangitis

Bacterial cholangitis has been described as the presenting symptom in approximately 6% of patients diagnosed with PSC.[11] Development of bacterial cholangitis is considered uncommon in the absence of prior biliary tree manipulation.[57] If symptoms of cholangitis develop, imaging to rule out choledocholithiasis or a dominant stricture is appropriate. Treatment may include antibiotic therapy with or without endoscopic intervention depending on probable cause. Less commonly, patients with PSC will require long-term prophylactic antibiotics. For those with intractable cholangitis, liver transplantation may be advisable.[58]

Osteoporosis

Metabolic bone disease is a relatively common complication of cirrhosis.[59] For patients with cholestatic liver disease, osteoporosis has been reported in up to 60%.[60] In a study of 81 patients, those with PSC had a lower bone mineral densitometry in their lumbar spine than their age- and sex-matched controls.[61] As such, screening for the condition with dual-energy x-ray absorptiometry is recommended at baseline with follow-up in 2 to 4 years, depending on the results.

The pathophysiology of metabolic bone disease in this setting is not well-understood. The risk of osteoporosis is increased with advanced age, female gender, low body weight, and in the setting of long-standing IBD. Replacement of vitamin D if deficiencies are known, along with use of calcium is recommended, as is weight-bearing exercise. Oral bisphosphonates may also be considered.[62]

Fat-Soluble Vitamin Deficiency

Patients with cholestatic liver disease are at an increased risk of fat-soluble vitamin deficiencies and malabsorption of nutrients owing to the diminished amount of bile salts in the intestine. Fat-soluble vitamin deficiency is more common in the setting of advanced stage liver disease than it is in early stage disease.[63] For patients with advanced staged disease, evaluation for vitamin D deficiency should be performed on an annual basis. If deficiency is noted, 50,000 U of water-soluble vitamin D provided twice weekly for 12 weeks is usually sufficient to correct the deficiency. Once a normal serum vitamin D level is achieved, a maintenance dose of 1000 IU/d is appropriate. Vitamin A deficiency is less common. Vitamin A levels when low should be replaced with 25,000 U 2 to 3 times per week. The adequacy of replacement therapy should be assessed with follow-up testing as excessive vitamin A has been associated with hepatotoxicity. Vitamin E may also be assessed and treated with replacement therapy if deficient, usually 800 to 1000 IU/d. Vitamin K levels are often most practically assessed by monitoring the prothrombin time. If prolonged or if the International Normalized Ratio is excessively elevated, 5 mg of vitamin K may be provided, particularly in the event invasive procedures are needed.

Portal Hypertension

PSC may progress to cirrhosis putting a patient at risk for portal hypertension. The mechanism whereby this occurs is not unique to PSC, but is consistent with all liver disease that progress to cirrhosis. That said, portal hypertension can be present in patients with PSC who do not have cirrhosis, although this is rare.[58]

The platelet level is a predictor of the presence of esophageal varices for patients with PSC and cirrhosis.[64] For most patients, use of nonselective beta-blockers as the primary prophylaxis is appropriate when small esophageal varices are known.

For patients who have had a variceal bleed, serial band ligation via upper gastrointestinal endoscopy is appropriate.[65]

Patients with portal hypertension may develop ascites. Management includes sodium restriction not to exceed 2 g/d in addition to diuretics, as needed. For most patients, combination therapy with a loop diuretic, such as furosemide, and an aldosterone agonist, such as spironolactone, is recommended. Treatment of hepatic encephalopathy typically includes use of lactulose, a synthetic disaccharide, by mouth or via nasogastric tube titrated to ensure 3 to 4 soft stools per day. Use of rifaximin, 550 mg twice daily, may also be added.

WHAT ARE THE INDICATIONS AND TIMING FOR LIVER TRANSPLANTATION FOR MY PATIENT WITH PRIMARY SCLEROSING CHOLANGITIS?

Approximately 40% of patients with PSC will eventually require liver transplantation.[10] Patients diagnosed with PSC may be considered for liver transplantation when they develop evidence of decompensated cirrhosis. Survival benefit is evident when the Model for End-Stage Liver Disease score exceeds 15.[66] The Model for End-Stage Liver Disease is calculated using the patient's bilirubin, International Normalized Ratios, and serum creatinine, which in concert measure the degree of hepatic dysfunction.

The 5-year survival for patients with PSC who have undergone liver transplantation with a deceased donor organ is 80% to 85%.[67,68] Patients who experience disease-related complications such as refractory pruritus or recurrent cholangitis are increasingly considering living donation rather than waiting for a deceased donor. Outcomes for patients who undergo living donor transplantation are similar or improved when compared with those who undergo transplant with a deceased donor organ.[69]

Patients who develop evidence of CCA may be candidates for liver transplantation through exception criteria granted by the United Network for Organ Sharing. This was previously considered an absolute contraindication; however, now patients with unresectable, early stage perihilar CCA measuring 3 cm or less in diameter without evidence of metastatic disease may be considered.[9] These patients receive neoadjuvant therapy with external beam radiation, radiosensitizing chemotherapy, endoscopic brachytherapy, and oral capecitabine before exploratory laparotomy to confirm candidacy before transplantation.[70]

Recurrence of PSC after liver transplantation occurs in perhaps 20% to 25% of patients after 10 years.[9,68] Management of these patients may include retransplantation, if indicated.

SUMMARY

PSC is a rare biliary tract disease that can lead to decreased quality of life, as well as end-stage liver disease and liver transplantation. Diagnosing patients with this condition may be challenging and requires keen diagnostic acumen. Ongoing management may include investigational therapies in addition to endoscopic interventions, as needed. Routine surveillance owing to the increased risk of hepatobiliary malignancy is necessary. The majority of patients with PSC have concurrent IBD. These patients have a significantly increased risk of colorectal carcinoma and heightened surveillance is recommended.

REFERENCES

1. Tabibian JH, Lindor KD. Primary sclerosing cholangitis: a review and update on therapeutic developments. Expert Rev Gastroenterol Hepatol 2013;7(2):103–14.

2. Levy C, Lindor KD. Primary sclerosing cholangitis: epidemiology, natural history, and prognosis. Semin Liver Dis 2006;26(1):22–30.
3. Hirschfield GM, Karlsen TH, Lindor KD, et al. Primary sclerosing cholangitis. Lancet 2013;382(9904):1587–99.
4. Lindor KD, Kowdley KV, Harrison ME, American College of Gastroenterology. ACG clinical guideline: primary sclerosing cholangitis. Am J Gastroenterol 2015;110(5):646–59 [quiz: 60].
5. Bambha K, Kim WR, Talwalkar J, et al. Incidence, clinical spectrum, and outcomes of primary sclerosing cholangitis in a United States community. Gastroenterology 2003;125(5):1364–9.
6. Lindkvist B, Benito de Valle M, Gullberg B, et al. Incidence and prevalence of primary sclerosing cholangitis in a defined adult population in Sweden. Hepatology 2010;52(2):571–7.
7. Boonstra K, Beuers U, Ponsioen CY. Epidemiology of primary sclerosing cholangitis and primary biliary cirrhosis: a systematic review. J Hepatol 2012;56(5):1181–8.
8. Molodecky NA, Kareemi H, Parab R, et al. Incidence of primary sclerosing cholangitis: a systematic review and meta-analysis. Hepatology 2011;53(5):1590–9.
9. Chapman R, Fevery J, Kalloo A, et al. Diagnosis and management of primary sclerosing cholangitis. Hepatology 2010;51(2):660–78.
10. Tischendorf JJ, Hecker H, Kruger M, et al. Characterization, outcome, and prognosis in 273 patients with primary sclerosing cholangitis: a single center study. Am J Gastroenterol 2007;102(1):107–14.
11. Kaplan GG, Laupland KB, Butzner D, et al. The burden of large and small duct primary sclerosing cholangitis in adults and children: a population-based analysis. Am J Gastroenterol 2007;102(5):1042–9.
12. Terjung B, Worman HJ. Anti-neutrophil antibodies in primary sclerosing cholangitis. Best Pract Res Clin Gastroenterol 2001;15(4):629–42.
13. Hov JR, Boberg KM, Taraldsrud E, et al. Antineutrophil antibodies define clinical and genetic subgroups in primary sclerosing cholangitis. Liver Int 2017;37(3):458–65.
14. MacCarty RL, LaRusso NF, Wiesner RH, et al. Primary sclerosing cholangitis: findings on cholangiography and pancreatography. Radiology 1983;149(1):39–44.
15. Stiehl A, Rudolph G, Kloters-Plachky P, et al. Development of dominant bile duct stenoses in patients with primary sclerosing cholangitis treated with ursodeoxycholic acid: outcome after endoscopic treatment. J Hepatol 2002;36(2):151–6.
16. Weber A, von Weyhern C, Fend F, et al. Endoscopic transpapillary brush cytology and forceps biopsy in patients with hilar cholangiocarcinoma. World J Gastroenterol 2008;14(7):1097–101.
17. Angulo P, Maor-Kendler Y, Lindor KD. Small-duct primary sclerosing cholangitis: a long-term follow-up study. Hepatology 2002;35(6):1494–500.
18. Bjornsson E, Boberg KM, Cullen S, et al. Patients with small duct primary sclerosing cholangitis have a favourable long term prognosis. Gut 2002;51(5):731–5.
19. Bjornsson E, Olsson R, Bergquist A, et al. The natural history of small-duct primary sclerosing cholangitis. Gastroenterology 2008;134(4):975–80.
20. Feldstein AE, Perrault J, El-Youssif M, et al. Primary sclerosing cholangitis in children: a long-term follow-up study. Hepatology 2003;38(1):210–7.
21. Kaya M, Angulo P, Lindor KD. Overlap of autoimmune hepatitis and primary sclerosing cholangitis: an evaluation of a modified scoring system. J Hepatol 2000;33(4):537–42.

22. Lee YM, Kaplan MM. Management of primary sclerosing cholangitis. Am J Gastroenterol 2002;97(3):528–34.

23. Shi J, Li Z, Zeng X, et al. Ursodeoxycholic acid in primary sclerosing cholangitis: meta-analysis of randomized controlled trials. Hepatol Res 2009;39(9):865–73.

24. Triantos CK, Koukias NM, Nikolopoulou VN, et al. Meta-analysis: ursodeoxycholic acid for primary sclerosing cholangitis. Aliment Pharmacol Ther 2011;34(8): 901–10.

25. Stanich PP, Bjornsson E, Gossard AA, et al. Alkaline phosphatase normalization is associated with better prognosis in primary sclerosing cholangitis. Dig Liver Dis 2011;43(4):309–13.

26. Lindstrom L, Hultcrantz R, Boberg KM, et al. Association between reduced levels of alkaline phosphatase and survival times of patients with primary sclerosing cholangitis. Clin Gastroenterol Hepatol 2013;11(7):841–6.

27. Lazaridis KN, LaRusso NF. Primary sclerosing cholangitis. N Engl J Med 2016; 375(25):2501–2.

28. Wunsch E, Trottier J, Milkiewicz M, et al. Prospective evaluation of ursodeoxycholic acid withdrawal in patients with primary sclerosing cholangitis. Hepatology 2014;60(3):931–40.

29. Schramm C, Schirmacher P, Helmreich-Becker I, et al. Combined therapy with azathioprine, prednisolone, and ursodiol in patients with primary sclerosing cholangitis. A case series. Ann Intern Med 1999;131(12):943–6.

30. Angulo P, Batts KP, Jorgensen RA, et al. Oral budesonide in the treatment of primary sclerosing cholangitis. Am J Gastroenterol 2000;95(9):2333–7.

31. Cullen SN, Chapman RW. Review article: current management of primary sclerosing cholangitis. Aliment Pharmacol Ther 2005;21(8):933–48.

32. Davies YK, Cox KM, Abdullah BA, et al. Long-term treatment of primary sclerosing cholangitis in children with oral vancomycin: an immunomodulating antibiotic. J Pediatr Gastroenterol Nutr 2008;47(1):61–7.

33. Rahimpour S, Nasiri-Toosi M, Khalili H, et al. A triple blinded, randomized, placebo-controlled clinical trial to evaluate the efficacy and safety of oral vancomycin in primary sclerosing cholangitis: a pilot study. J Gastrointest Liver Dis 2016;25(4):457–64.

34. Boonstra K, Weersma RK, van Erpecum KJ, et al. Population-based epidemiology, malignancy risk, and outcome of primary sclerosing cholangitis. Hepatology 2013;58(6):2045–55.

35. Bergquist A, Ekbom A, Olsson R, et al. Hepatic and extrahepatic malignancies in primary sclerosing cholangitis. J Hepatol 2002;36(3):321–7.

36. Rizvi S, Eaton JE, Gores GJ. Primary sclerosing cholangitis as a premalignant biliary tract disease: surveillance and management. Clin Gastroenterol Hepatol 2015;13(12):2152–65.

37. Harnois DM, Gores GJ, Ludwig J, et al. Are patients with cirrhotic stage primary sclerosing cholangitis at risk for the development of hepatocellular cancer? J Hepatol 1997;27(3):512–6.

38. Zenouzi R, Weismuller TJ, Hubener P, et al. Low risk of hepatocellular carcinoma in patients with primary sclerosing cholangitis with cirrhosis. Clin Gastroenterol Hepatol 2014;12(10):1733–8.

39. Razumilava N, Gores GJ, Lindor KD. Cancer surveillance in patients with primary sclerosing cholangitis. Hepatology 2011;54(5):1842–52.

40. Charatcharoenwitthaya P, Enders FB, Halling KC, et al. Utility of serum tumor markers, imaging, and biliary cytology for detecting cholangiocarcinoma in primary sclerosing cholangitis. Hepatology 2008;48(4):1106–17.

41. Levy C, Lymp J, Angulo P, et al. The value of serum CA 19-9 in predicting cholangiocarcinomas in patients with primary sclerosing cholangitis. Dig Dis Sci 2005;50(9):1734–40.

42. Barr Fritcher EG, Voss JS, Jenkins SM, et al. Primary sclerosing cholangitis with equivocal cytology: fluorescence in situ hybridization and serum CA 19-9 predict risk of malignancy. Cancer Cytopathol 2013;121(12):708–17.

43. Kipp BR, Stadheim LM, Halling SA, et al. A comparison of routine cytology and fluorescence in situ hybridization for the detection of malignant bile duct strictures. Am J Gastroenterol 2004;99(9):1675–81.

44. Bangarulingam SY, Bjornsson E, Enders F, et al. Long-term outcomes of positive fluorescence in situ hybridization tests in primary sclerosing cholangitis. Hepatology 2010;51(1):174–80.

45. Said K, Glaumann H, Bergquist A. Gallbladder disease in patients with primary sclerosing cholangitis. J Hepatol 2008;48(4):598–605.

46. Buckles DC, Lindor KD, Larusso NF, et al. In primary sclerosing cholangitis, gallbladder polyps are frequently malignant. Am J Gastroenterol 2002;97(5): 1138–42.

47. Eaton JE, Thackeray EW, Lindor KD. Likelihood of malignancy in gallbladder polyps and outcomes following cholecystectomy in primary sclerosing cholangitis. Am J Gastroenterol 2012;107(3):431–9.

48. Soetikno RM, Lin OS, Heidenreich PA, et al. Increased risk of colorectal neoplasia in patients with primary sclerosing cholangitis and ulcerative colitis: a meta-analysis. Gastrointest Endosc 2002;56(1):48–54.

49. Khaderi SA, Sussman NL. Screening for malignancy in primary sclerosing cholangitis (PSC). Curr Gastroenterol Rep 2015;17(4):17.

50. Stiehl A. Primary sclerosing cholangitis: the role of endoscopic therapy. Semin Liver Dis 2006;26(1):62–8.

51. Johnson GK, Saeian K, Geenen JE. Primary sclerosing cholangitis treated by endoscopic biliary dilation: review and long-term follow-up evaluation. Curr Gastroenterol Rep 2006;8(2):147–55.

52. Kaya M, Petersen BT, Angulo P, et al. Balloon dilation compared to stenting of dominant strictures in primary sclerosing cholangitis. Am J Gastroenterol 2001; 96(4):1059–66.

53. van Milligen de Wit AW, Rauws EA, van Bracht J, et al. Lack of complications following short-term stent therapy for extrahepatic bile duct strictures in primary sclerosing cholangitis. Gastrointest Endosc 1997;46(4):344–7.

54. Choi SH, Gwon DI, Ko GY, et al. Hepatic arterial injuries in 3110 patients following percutaneous transhepatic biliary drainage. Radiology 2011;261(3):969–75.

55. Savader SJ, Trerotola SO, Merine DS, et al. Hemobilia after percutaneous transhepatic biliary drainage: treatment with transcatheter embolotherapy. J Vasc Interv Radiol 1992;3(2):345–52.

56. Ginat D, Saad WE, Davies MG, et al. Incidence of cholangitis and sepsis associated with percutaneous transhepatic biliary drain cholangiography and exchange: a comparison between liver transplant and native liver patients. AJR Am J Roentgenol 2011;196(1):W73–7.

57. Lindor KD, Wiesner RH, MacCarty RL, et al. Advances in primary sclerosing cholangitis. Am J Med 1990;89(1):73–80.

58. Abraham SC, Kamath PS, Eghtesad B, et al. Liver transplantation in precirrhotic biliary tract disease: portal hypertension is frequently associated with nodular regenerative hyperplasia and obliterative portal venopathy. Am J Surg Pathol 2006;30(11):1454–61.

59. Sokhi RP, Anantharaju A, Kondaveeti R, et al. Bone mineral density among cirrhotic patients awaiting liver transplantation. Liver Transpl 2004;10(5):648–53.
60. Gasser RW. Cholestasis and metabolic bone disease - a clinical review. Wien Med Wochenschr 2008;158(19–20):553–7.
61. Angulo P, Therneau TM, Jorgensen A, et al. Bone disease in patients with primary sclerosing cholangitis: prevalence, severity and prediction of progression. J Hepatol 1998;29(5):729–35.
62. Collier J. Bone disorders in chronic liver disease. Hepatology 2007;46(4):1271–8.
63. Jorgensen RA, Lindor KD, Sartin JS, et al. Serum lipid and fat-soluble vitamin levels in primary sclerosing cholangitis. J Clin Gastroenterol 1995;20(3):215–9.
64. Zein CO, Lindor KD, Angulo P. Prevalence and predictors of esophageal varices in patients with primary sclerosing cholangitis. Hepatology 2004;39(1):204–10.
65. Garcia-Tsao G, Sanyal AJ, Grace ND, et al, Practice Guidelines Committee of American Association for Study of Liver Diseases, Practice Parameters Committee of American College of Gastroenterology. Prevention and management of gastroesophageal varices and variceal hemorrhage in cirrhosis. Hepatology 2007;46(3):922–38.
66. Merion RM, Schaubel DE, Dykstra DM, et al. The survival benefit of liver transplantation. Am J Transplant 2005;5(2):307–13.
67. Graziadei IW, Wiesner RH, Marotta PJ, et al. Long-term results of patients undergoing liver transplantation for primary sclerosing cholangitis. Hepatology 1999;30(5):1121–7.
68. Fosby B, Karlsen TH, Melum E. Recurrence and rejection in liver transplantation for primary sclerosing cholangitis. World J Gastroenterol 2012;18(1):1–15.
69. Kashyap R, Safadjou S, Chen R, et al. Living donor and deceased donor liver transplantation for autoimmune and cholestatic liver diseases–an analysis of the UNOS database. J Gastrointest Surg 2010;14(9):1362–9.
70. Darwish Murad S, Kim WR, Harnois DM, et al. Efficacy of neoadjuvant chemoradiation, followed by liver transplantation, for perihilar cholangiocarcinoma at 12 US centers. Gastroenterology 2012;143(1):88–98.e3 [quiz: e14].

Treatment Strategies for Nonalcoholic Fatty Liver Disease and Nonalcoholic Steatohepatitis

Pegah Golabi, MD[a], Haley Bush, MSPH[a],
Zobair M. Younossi, MD, MPH[a,b,*]

KEYWORDS

- NAFLD • NASH • Treatment • Clinical trials • Nonantifibrotics

KEY POINTS

- Nonalcoholic fatty liver disease (NAFLD) and nonalcoholic steatohepatitis (NASH) have been increasingly recognized as global health problems.
- Treatment strategies have been focusing on patients with more advanced liver disease.
- Lifestyle modification and vitamin E treatment are effective in the treatment of NAFLD; other treatment options are not approved and not based on strong evidence.
- New agents are mainly targeting oxidative stress, inflammation, apoptosis, peroxisome proliferator-activated receptor family, insulin resistance, bile acid metabolism, farnesoid X receptor, and lipid metabolism.
- Phase II and III studies are underway, targeting different points of NAFLD and NASH pathogenesis, which will help in developing personalized treatment options.

INTRODUCTION

Nonalcoholic fatty liver disease (NAFLD) is one of the leading causes of chronic liver disease in adults.[1,2] With the increasing obesity rates all over the world, the global prevalence of NAFLD has increased sharply and now it is affecting one-fourth of the general population in the United States and the rest of the world.[3]

Disclosure Statement: The authors have nothing to disclose.
[a] Betty and Guy Beatty Center for Integrated Research, Inova Health System, Inova Fairfax Hospital, Claude Moore Health Education and Research Building, 3rd Floor, 3300 Gallows Road, Falls Church, VA 22042, USA; [b] Department of Medicine, Center for Liver Disease, Inova Fairfax Hospital, Claude Moore Health Education and Research Building, 3rd Floor, 3300 Gallows Road, Falls Church, VA 22042, USA
* Corresponding author. Betty and Guy Beatty Center for Integrated Research, Inova Health System, Inova Fairfax Hospital, Claude Moore Health Education and Research Building, 3rd Floor, 3300 Gallows Road, Falls Church, VA 22042.
E-mail address: Zobair.Younossi@inova.org

Clin Liver Dis 21 (2017) 739–753
http://dx.doi.org/10.1016/j.cld.2017.06.010
1089-3261/17/© 2017 Elsevier Inc. All rights reserved.

liver.theclinics.com

NAFLD covers a wide variety of conditions, from nonalcoholic steatohepatitis (NASH) to non-NASH NAFLD which encompasses steatosis alone. Although it is still debated, NASH subjects are primarily at an increased risk of developing fibrosis, cirrhosis, and hepatocellular carcinoma.[4] In fact, NASH is currently the second most common indication for liver transplantation and estimated to be the leading indication in the next 1 to 2 decades.[5] NAFLD is correlated intricately with insulin resistance and obesity, and because of strong associations with type 2 diabetes, hypertension, and dyslipidemia, it has been regarded as the hepatic manifestation of the metabolic syndrome.[3] Some NAFLD subjects are lean.[6] In fact, the majority of NAFLD subjects from rural areas of India and potentially other Asian countries have lean NAFLD.[7] In addition to the clinical impact, NAFLD has important economic impact on the society.[8] Finally, NAFLD and its advanced stages impairs patients' health-related quality of life, with a negative impact on patients' experience.[9]

Pathophysiologic Target for the Treatment of Nonalcoholic Steatohepatitis

Given its potentially progressive nature, NASH subjects are candidates for treatment protocols. In fact, the most appropriate subjects with NASH that should be the focus of clinical trials are those NASH subjects with significant fibrosis.[10] In this context, treatment strategies have targeted the accumulation of fat in the liver, or pathways that lead to liver cell injury and ultimately hepatic fibrosis. Additionally, other treatment strategies have targeted hepatic fibrosis with agents that have potential antifibrotic effects.[11]

Accumulation of lipid in hepatocytes causes fatty infiltration and there are various pathways that can lead to hepatic steatosis. These pathways include increased free fatty acid supply to hepatocytes as a major mechanism for steatosis. In fact, this process can occur either from increased intake of fat in the diet or increased lipolysis in the adipose tissue leading to higher amounts of lipids transferring to liver as well as increased de novo hepatic lipogenesis, decreased free fatty acid oxidation, and decreased very low density lipoprotein secretion in the liver.[12] Triglycerides are the major type of lipids stored in the liver of patients with NAFLD. The accumulation of triglycerides in hepatocytes is not always considered a pathologic condition. However, the accumulation of free fatty acids, especially in the mitochondria, may lead to the formation of reactive oxygen species and tumor necrosis factor (TNF)-α, which can further mediate liver damage.[13] These factors are the important elements of "multiple hit" hypothesis, which has been used to explain the pathogenesis of progression of NAFLD. According to this theory, insulin resistance represents the first hit. Because of the hyperinsulinemia, hepatic lipogenesis increases and lipolysis in the adipose tissue cannot be suppressed properly, both of which cause an increased efflux of free fatty acids from the adipose tissue to liver. In this context, hepatocytes become more susceptible to further harmful events, which represents the other multiple hits, including oxidative stress from reactive oxygen species, the TNF-α pathway, activation of the transforming growth factor-β pathway (a profibrogenic event), increased and dysregulated hepatocyte apoptosis, stellate cell activation, and dysregulation of adipocytokines.[14] All these insults result in recruitment of immune cells to damaged areas, which leads to further hepatocyte injury and worsening of inflammation.

Owing to the various mechanisms that contribute to the development of NAFLD and NASH, the number of strategies and treatment targets continue to grow. Although the first step in NAFLD treatment has been lifestyle modification with diet and exercise, other promising pharmacologic agents are emerging. **Table 1** shows the currently available effective treatment options for NAFLD and NASH.

Table 1
Effective treatment options for nonalcoholic fatty liver disease and NASH

Option	Role	Effect	Notes
Diet modification	Various dietary recommendations available Mediterranean diet was shown to have better cardiovascular outcomes	5%–10% weight loss achievable with diet modification Significant improvements in activity score and inflammation when losing 7% of body weight	Rapid weight loss was associated with worsening hepatic fibrosis and inflammation
Physical activity	Aerobic or resistance, 3–4 times a week, at 20–40 minutes per session, at moderate intensity	Reduction in intrahepatic fat content Augmentation of fat mobilization from liver	Either aerobic or resistance exercise is ideal for fat mobilization from the liver In most cases, increased physical activity is combined with a healthier diet
Vitamin E	Antioxidant Free radical scavenger	Reduction in serum aminotransferase levels Improvement in lobular inflammation and hepatocyte ballooning	Only medication recommended by guidelines (Others depend on strong evidence)
Pentoxifylline	Nonspecific phosphodiesterase inhibitor Decreases TNF-α gene transcription	Improved steatosis, lobular inflammation and fibrosis	
Pioglitazone	PPAR-γ agonist	Decreasing lobular inflammation in NASH	PIVENS study did not reach primary endpoint Data on hepatic fibrosis have been inconsistent
Saroglitazar	PPAR-α/γ agonist	Management of diabetic dyslipidemia	PRESS V showed benefit on diabetic dyslipidemia A phase IIa study is underway for histologic findings
Elafibranor	PPAR-α/δ agonist	Resolution of NASH without fibrosis worsening	GOLDEN-505 study did not meet the predefined end point in the intention-to-treat group Resolution of NASH significant in the 120 mg group

(continued on next page)

Table 1 (continued)			
Option	Role	Effect	Notes
Liraglutide Exenatide	GLP-1 agonist	Improving insulin sensitivity, increasing β-oxidation of free fatty acids in the hepatocytes, resolution of NASH	LEAN study showed improvement in liver histology
Obeticholic acid	Modified bile acid	Increase in glucose-stimulated insulin secretion Inhibition of hepatic lipid synthesis Increased lipid uptake by adipocytes	FLINT study showed histologic improvement in patients treated with obeticholic acid
Aramchol	Synthetic lipid SCD-1 inhibitor	Safe and effective in reducing hepatic fat content	

Abbreviations: GLP-1, glucagon-like peptide 1; NASH, nonalcoholic steatohepatitis; PPAR, peroxisome proliferator-activated receptor; TNF-α, tumor necrosis factor-α.

Lifestyle Modification: Diet and Exercise

Currently, lifestyle modification is the accepted first line treatment for patients with NAFLD and NASH. However, lifestyle modification is a general term and the components often differ according to clinical situation. When health care providers recommend lifestyle changes for the treatment of NAFLD, most of the time it refers to sustained weight loss and an increase in the amount of exercise the patient does.[15]

In the last decades, several dietary models have been proposed as ideal for the management of NAFLD. Among those recommendations, the most emphasized diet has been the Mediterranean diet. In fact, the Mediterranean diet was first discovered in the 1960s and was recognized as a healthy diet, effective in reducing the risk of cardiovascular diseases and cancer.[16] Its beneficial effects in patients with NAFLD have been reported in multiple studies.[17,18] To show the effect of weight loss on NAFLD, Promrat and colleagues[19] conducted a randomized, controlled trial and reported that patients who followed the lifestyle intervention had an average of 10% weight loss and patients who lost more than 7% of their body weight had significant improvements in activity score and inflammation. The speed of weight loss is also important because rapid weight loss has been periodically reported to worsen hepatic fibrosis and inflammation.[20]

Increased physical activity has also an independent potential to greatly benefit NAFLD patients. In fact, exercise has been documented to be an effective intervention for reducing intrahepatic lipid content by reducing hepatic lipogenesis and augmenting fat mobilization from the liver.[21] A recent systematic review demonstrated that either aerobic or resistance, 3 to 4 times a week, at 20 to 40 minutes per session, and at moderate intensity is ideal for fat mobilization from the liver in patients with NAFLD.[22] However, in most cases, increased physical activity is combined with a healthier diet, to boost the beneficial effect of each intervention.

Treatment Regimens Targeting Oxidative Stress, Inflammation, Apoptosis, and the Immune System

When lifestyle modification is not successful, or insufficient, clinicians may offer pharmacologic treatment that could potentially target one of the responsible mechanisms. As mentioned, reactive oxygen species and oxidative stress are key components in the pathophysiology of NAFLD, and agents against this oxidative stress may be used in the treatment of NAFLD. Vitamin E is a fat-soluble molecule, and is an antioxidant and protects cell membranes from oxidation. In fact, vitamin E works as a free radical scavenger and protects the major structural components of cell membranes, such as polyunsaturated fatty acids, from peroxidation.[23] Vitamin E was tried in patients with NAFLD, to suppress the hepatic inflammation by inactivating free radicals and suppressing lipid peroxidation.[24] In fact, the PIVENS trial (Pioglitazone vs Vitamin E vs Placebo for Treatment of Non-Diabetic Patients With Nonalcoholic Steatohepatitis) compared the effect of pioglitazone and vitamin E with placebo among nondiabetic patients with biopsy-proven NASH. This study showed that vitamin E reduced serum aminotransferase levels and improved lobular inflammation better than placebo among patients with NASH.[25] Another study, the TONIC trial (Treatment of Nonalcoholic Fatty Liver Disease in Children), evaluated the impact of vitamin E or metformin in children and adolescents with NAFLD. This study showed that, compared with the placebo group, there was a significant improvement in hepatocellular ballooning scores and NAFLD activity scores in the vitamin E group, as well as the rate of NASH resolution.[26] Based on these findings, current guidelines recommend the use of vitamin E for patients with NASH.[15] Most studies suggest that vitamin E supplementation in doses of 100 to 400 IU/d is safe for most patients. In fact, in 2017, vitamin E is the only treatment that is, recommended by the American Association for the Study of Liver Diseases guidelines for treatment of patients with biopsy-proven NASH without diabetes and cirrhosis.[27,28]

Outside vitamin E, no other pharmacologic intervention has been recommended. In fact, although other treatment regimens have been offered in the clinical setting, it is important to note that these regimens are not approved and the recommendations are not based on strong evidence.

In this context, TNF-α has been implicated in the pathogenesis of NASH by promoting inflammation, apoptosis, and fibrosis, as well as by interfering with the insulin signaling transduction pathway.[29] Pentoxifylline (PTX) is a methylxanthine derivative that works as a nonspecific phosphodiesterase inhibitor and decreases TNF-α gene transcription. Zein and colleagues[30] conducted a placebo-controlled randomized clinical trial with 55 patients with biopsy-proven NASH to determine the effects of PTX on histologic features of NASH. After 1 year, PTX significantly improved steatosis, lobular inflammation, and liver fibrosis in comparison with placebo, but no significant effects in hepatocellular ballooning were observed. A metaanalysis by Du and colleagues[31] showed that PTX treatment can lower liver enzymes, improve NAFLD Activity Score and lobular inflammation. Despite these data, a robust well-designed clinical trial to assess the efficacy of PTX in subjects with NASH is not available and currently this treatment cannot be routinely recommended to treat NASH.

Another pathway that can potentially contribute to the pathogenesis of NASH is related to the inflammatory milieu. In this context, the activation of Kupffer cells and proinflammatory macrophages may play a key role in the activation of stellate cells triggering fibrogenic pathways.[32] In these intercellular signaling pathways, CCR2 and CCR5 may play an important role and could be the target of treatment for NASH. Furthermore, therapeutic agents that could inhibit these 2 receptors may provide an effective treatment option for patients with NASH. In this context, cenicriviroc is an immunomodulatory agent that can inhibit both CCR2 and CCR5. Lefebvre and colleagues[33] demonstrated the potent antiinflammatory and antifibrotic activities of cenicriviroc in a range of animal fibrosis models. The CENTAUR study (Efficacy and Safety Study of Cenicriviroc for the Treatment of NASH in Adult Subjects With Liver Fibrosis) is a phase IIb, randomized, double-blind, placebo-controlled, multinational study aiming to assess the effects of cenicriviroc on histologic improvement and NASH resolution without worsening of fibrosis, among noncirrhotic patients with NASH.[34] The preliminary analysis of a phase II clinical trial with this agent showed that, despite an inability to meet the primary outcome of NASH resolution, there was significant reduction in fibrosis.[35] A large phase III clinical trial of this agent for treatment of NASH is currently being designed.[36] **Table 2** summarizes the clinical trials currently underway for treatment of NASH.

Another important pathway that can result in apoptosis and development of fibrosis is the activation of apoptosis signal-regulating kinase 1. Apoptosis signal-regulating kinase 1 activation results in production of inflammatory cytokines, chemokines, expression of matrix remodeling genes, and promotion of apoptotic cell death. Selonsertib is an apoptosis signal-regulating kinase 1 inhibitor and has been assessed in a phase II clinical trial. The results of this study showed potential efficacy and a good safety profile.[37] In fact, the efficacy of these regimens is being assessed in 2 large phase III clinical trials (STELLAR 3 and 4 [STELLAR-Rosuvastatin vs. Atorvastatin, Pravastatin, Simvastatin Across Dose Ranges]) for patients with NASH with advanced fibrosis (stage 3 and stage 4).

Finally, lipopolysaccharides and endogenous gut-derived bacterial endotoxins have been suggested to play a role in NASH. For this reason, recent clinical trials are also focusing on immunomodulators that can potential impact this pathway. Adar and colleagues[38] reported that oral administration of IgG-enhanced colostrum was able to reduce the triglyceride level both in the serum and also in the liver. Hyperimmune bovine colostrum, which acts as an inductor of regulatory T cells, is currently being studied in a phase IIa trial. The primary endpoint of the study is the change in hepatic fat content in patients with NASH.

Peroxisome Proliferator-activated Receptors Family

Peroxisome proliferator-activated receptors (PPAR) are ligand-activated transcription factors that regulate genes important in cell differentiation, as well as metabolic processes, including glucose and lipid homeostasis. PPARs are a family of ligand-activated nuclear hormone receptors, which means that, after interaction with specific ligands, nuclear receptors are translocated to the nucleus and regulate gene expression.[39] There are 3 isoforms in the PPAR family: PPAR-α, PPAR-β/δ, and PPAR-γ, which differ in tissue distribution and physiologic effects.

Because insulin resistance is a primary characteristic of NAFLD and NASH, insulin sensitizers have been used in treatment. The thiazolidinediones (TZDs), pioglitazone and rosiglitazone, modulate insulin sensitivity via PPAR-γ signaling.[40] Current literature suggests that patients with NASH who were treated with TZDs may show improvement of hepatosteatosis, lobular inflammation, and hepatocyte ballooning, but the data on hepatic fibrosis have been inconsistent. In fact, the PIVENS trial, a randomized, placebo-controlled clinical trial of pioglitazone in nondiabetics with NASH, did not achieve its primary endpoint.[25] Nevertheless, a recent metaanalysis by He and colleagues[41] reported that both the overall and subgroup analyses can reveal some benefit of TZDs by decreasing lobular inflammation in NASH. In the

Table 2
Current clinical trials for treatment of nonalcoholic steatohepatitis

Agent	Mechanism	Trials
Cenicriviroc	CCR2 and CCR5 receptors inhibitor Antifibrotic activities on animal model	CENTUAR trial Histologic improvement in NAS score with no concurrent worsening of fibrosis stage Improvement in fibrosis by at least 1 stage (NASH CRN system) with no worsening of steatohepatitis
Selonsertib	ASK1 inhibitor	STELLAR 3 and 4 trials assessing efficacy on NASH with advanced fibrosis
Hyperimmune bovine colostrum	Inducer of regulatory T cells	A phase IIa trial is assessing the effect of this medication on hepatic fat content
MSDC-0602K	mTOR-modulating insulin sensitizer	A phase IIa trial is assessing the effect in patients with NASH
Elafibranor	PPARα/δ agonist	RESOLVE-IT trial assessing long-term evaluation of this medication on stage 1–3 fibrosis in NASH
IVA337	Pan PPAR (α, δ, γ) agonist	NATIVE trial evaluating effect on liver histology among patients with NASH
OCA	Modified bile acid	REGENERATE trial assessing long term effects of OCA on NASH fibrosis
NGM282	Recombinant FGF 19 agonist	A phase IIa trial is assessing effect on hepatic fat content
BMS-986036	Recombinant FGF 21 agonist	A phase IIa trial is assessing effect on hepatic fat content
Volixibat	ASBT inhibitor	A phase IIa trial is assessing improvement in NAS score without worsening fibrosis
MGL-3196	THR-β agonist	A phase IIa trial is assessing the change in the hepatic fat content
GS-0976	Acetyl-CoA carboxylase inhibitor	A phase IIa trial is assessing effect on patients with NASH
GS-0976 & GS-9674	Acetyl-CoA carboxylase inhibitor + FXR agonist	A phase IIa trial is assessing effect on patients with NASH
JKB-121	Nonselective opioid antagonist	A phase IIa trial is assessing effect on patients with NASH

Abbreviations: ASBT, apical sodium-dependent bile acid transporter; ASK1, apoptosis signal-regulating kinase 1; CoA, coenzyme A; CRN, Clinical Research Network; FGF, fibroblast growth factor; FXR, farnesoid X receptor; mTOR, mammalian target of rapamycin; NAFLD, nonalcoholic fatty live disease; NAS, NAFLD Activity Score; OCA, obeticholic acid; THR, thyroid hormone receptor.

same study, overall analysis revealed improvement in hepatic fibrosis in TZD-treated patients, but this significance was not observed in the subgroup analysis.

Another agent, saroglitazar, is a dual PPAR-α/γ agonist and is shown to be an effective and safe therapeutic option for the management of diabetic dyslipidemia in the PRESS V study (Prospective Randomized Efficacy and Safety of Saroglitazar).[42] A phase IIa clinical trial is underway to evaluate the benefit of saroglitazar at a histologic level in patients with NASH. MSDC-0602 K is a newly developed TZD analogue that has a low affinity for activating PPAR-γ, but has similar insulin sensitizing properties as rosiglitazone does. It does not alter CD36 expression in the bone-reabsorptive cells, and thus does not increase osteoclast differentiation and number.[43] MSDC-0602K is currently being studied in a phase IIa study to assess its beneficial effect in patients with NASH.

Different from PPAR-γ, PPAR-α expression is relatively high in hepatocytes, enterocytes, and some vascular immune cell types like macrophages and monocytes.[44] In the liver, PPAR-α plays a crucial role by controlling lipid flux through the modulation of fatty acid transport and β-oxidation, hence improving plasma lipids by decreasing triglycerides and increasing high-density lipoprotein cholesterol. PPAR-α activation also inhibits some inflammatory genes and decreases the expression of acute phase response genes.[45] Similarly, PPAR-δ activity enhances fatty acid transportation and oxidation, improves glucose homeostasis, and exerts antiinflammatory activities on Kupffer cells. The GOLDEN-505 trial (Phase IIb Study to Evaluate the Efficacy and Safety of GFT505 Versus Placebo in Patients With Non-Alcoholic Steatohepatitis), a double-blind, placebo-controlled, randomized, international phase IIb trial, reported the potential impact of elafibranor, which is a dual PPAR-α/δ agonist, in patients with NASH without cirrhosis.[45] In the initial analysis, there was no difference between the 2 elafibranor groups (80 and 120 mg/d) and placebo group in achieving the study's primary outcome. Nevertheless, the authors reported that elafibranor at 120 mg/d was significantly superior to placebo in the post hoc analysis.[45] The RESOLVE-IT trial (Phase 3 Study to Evaluate the Efficacy and Safety of Elafibranor Versus Placebo in Patients With Nonalcoholic Steatohepatitis) is a large, randomized, placebo-controlled, double-blind, multicenter phase III study, planning to enroll around 2000 patients with NASH and stage 1 to 3 fibrosis, for the long-term evaluation of elafibranor in NASH.

IVA337 is a recently developed pan-PPAR agonist ($\alpha/\delta/\gamma$) that was studied in patients with systemic sclerosis for its effects on inflammation and fibrosis.[46] The NATIVE trial (NAsh Trial to Validate IVA337 Efficacy) is a phase IIa clinical trial, currently evaluating the effects of IVA337 on liver histology among patients with NASH.

Another group of medication in the PPAR family are fibrates, which are PPAR-α agonists, whose effects are mainly lowering high triglyceride levels, increasing high-density lipoprotein cholesterol, and lowering low-density lipoprotein cholesterol. They are mainly used in the treatment of hypertriglyceridemia, which is relatively common in patients with NAFLD, but has no significant benefit for the histologic changes seen in NAFLD and NASH.[47]

AGENTS AGAINST HYPERGLYCEMIA AND INSULIN RESISTANCE

Metformin was one of the initial medications used in the treatment of hyperglycemia and has known benefits regarding weight loss, improvement of insulin resistance, and even reducing the risk of hepatocellular carcinoma among patients with diabetes. Doycheva and colleagues[48] reported that adult patients who were able to lose weight and improve transaminase levels during metformin treatment showed improved hepatocyte ballooning in posttreatment liver biopsies. Nevertheless, the majority of studies assessing metformin for NASH do not show significant efficacy. Therefore, at the time of this writing, the use of metformin for treatment of NASH cannot be supported by published evidence.

Besides metformin, treatment of hyperglycemia includes many other pharmacologic agents, including sulfonylureas, TZDs, dipeptidyl peptidase 4 (DPP-4) inhibitors, sodium-glucose cotransporter 2 inhibitor, and glucagon-like peptide 1 (GLP-1) agonists, as well as different types of insulin. The detailed mechanisms of these medications is beyond the topic of this article; however, some of these drugs may have efficacy for treating NASH but require properly performed clinical trials.

Incretin-based therapies have emerged for the use of incretin system for the treatment of hyperglycemia in diabetic patients. Two classes of incretin therapies include DPP-4 inhibitors, which prevent the proteolytic breakdown and inactivation of GLP-1, and GLP-1 receptor agonists, which provide stimulation of the receptor by high concentration of ligands.[49] GLP-1 is a hormone that is secreted by L cells in the distal ileum within minutes after eating, and mainly regulates the amount of insulin that is secreted after food intake.[50] Aside from stimulating insulin secretion, GLP-1 has many other roles in the gastrointestinal tract, including inhibiting glucagon secretion, suppressing appetite, delaying gastric emptying, enhancing glucose uptake by the hepatocytes, and improving insulin sensitivity.[51] In hepatocytes, GLP-1 agonists cause an increase in PPAR-α and PPAR-γ expression, which results in increased β-oxidation of free fatty acids and disposition of lipids.

Carbone and colleagues[52] reported in their metaanalysis that GLP-1 agonists and DPP-4 inhibitors achieved significant improvements in serum alanine aminotransferase levels. Armstrong and colleagues[53] showed in the LEAN study (Liraglutide efficacy and action in non-alcoholic steatohepatitis), a phase II, multicenter, double-blinded, placebo-controlled, randomized clinical trial, that 48-week treatment with 1.8 mg liraglutide resulted in resolution of NASH in 39% of the participants in a repeat liver biopsy at the end of the treatment. Another study showed significant improvement in liver histology of a small proportion of diabetic patients who received exenatide for 28 weeks, but there were also high rates of gastrointestinal side effects.[54] However, in terms of DPP-4 inhibitors like sitagliptin and vildagliptin, further evidence must be generated from well-designed clinical trials before their efficacy and safety in NASH treatment can be determined.

Sodium-glucose transporter in the kidneys is another target for diabetes treatment and remogliflozin is a member of sodium-glucose transporter-2 inhibitors. Preclinical studies showed a decrease in the hepatic fat content and markers of oxidative stress, as well as reversal of insulin sensitivity and a decrease in alanine aminotransferase levels among diabetic patients receiving sodium-glucose cotransporter-2 inhibitors. This may be a potential pharmacologic agent for the treatment of NAFLD and NASH.[55]

Bile Acid Metabolism: Farnesoid X Receptor

Obeticholic acid (OCA) is a modified bile acid, derived from chenodeoxycholic acid, which is the natural ligand for the farnesoid X receptor (FXR). OCA increases glucose-stimulated insulin secretion, augments peripheral glucose uptake, inhibits hepatic lipid synthesis, and induces lipid uptake by adipocytes. In a multicenter, double-blind, placebo-controlled randomized clinical trial (FLINT [Farnesoid X nuclear receptor ligand obeticholic acid for non-cirrhotic, non-alcoholic steatohepatitis]), Neuschwander-Tetri and colleagues[56] reported on the efficacy of OCA in adult patients with biopsy-proven NASH. In this trial, patients were randomly assigned to receive either 25 mg of OCA or placebo for 72 weeks. The findings of the FLINT trial showed that patients who received OCA for 72 weeks had significantly higher histologic improvement rates than patients in the placebo arm. Treatment with OCA improved steatosis, hepatocellular ballooning, lobular inflammation, and decreased the severity of fibrosis. REGENERATE (Randomized Global Phase 3 Study to Evaluate the Impact on NASH With Fibrosis of Obeticholic Acid Treatment) is planned to be a double-blind, placebo-controlled, randomized, multicenter phase III trial to assess the long-term evaluation of OCA for NASH and fibrosis. This trial will enroll around 2000 patients with biopsy-proven NASH, ideally stage 2 or 3 fibrosis.

FXR is a nuclear receptor, expressed at high levels in liver, kidneys, and intestines.[57] FXR agonists lower hepatic triglycerides via the SREPB-1C pathway and decrease bile acid synthesis by shutting down the CYP7a1 enzyme. This enzyme converts cholesterol to bile acid, increases fatty acid oxidation, and decreases gluconeogenesis, portal pressure, and inflammation.[57]

Recent research has highlighted the role of FXR-dependent fibroblast growth factor 19 (FGF19) in the hepatic lipid metabolism. FGF19 is a member of FGF family, expressed in the intestines, and functions as an enterohepatic hormone. FGF19 acts on the liver, downregulates hepatic expression of CYP7a1, and decreases bile acid synthesis.[58] NGM282 is a recombinant FGF19 agonist that mainly binds to 2 different molecules, FGFR4 and FGFR1c. Therefore, it not only inhibits bile acid formation by blocking CYP7a1 enzyme, but it also improves insulin sensitization. NGM282 is currently being studied in a phase IIa trial with the primary endpoint being change in hepatic fat content among patients with NASH.[59]

Another member of FGF family, FGF21, is mostly produced in the liver, pancreas, muscle, and adipose tissues, where it improves insulin sensitivity and ameliorates hepatic steatosis.[60] In this context, BMS986036 is a recombinant FGF21 agonist, whose main activity is through the FGFR1c pathway, but is also has activity through FGFR2 and FGFR3. It primarily improves glycemic control by decreasing hepatic glucose production, increasing peripheral glucose turnover, increasing β cell preservation, correcting dyslipidemia (by increasing high-density lipoprotein cholesterol and decreasing low-density lipoprotein cholesterol and triglyceride levels), and has a possible weight loss effect. BMS986036 is also being studied in a phase IIa trial for its role in changing hepatic fat content in patients with NASH.[59]

Bile acid transporters belong to a solute carrier-10 family of integral membrane proteins and comprise multiple members including the apical sodium-dependent bile acid transporter and Na-taurocholate cotransporting polypeptide. Together, these 2 systems maintain the enterohepatic recycling of bile acids within the gastrointestinal tract and the liver, and play a critical role in cholesterol homeostasis.[61] For this reason, apical sodium-dependent bile acid transporter inhibition has emerged as a valuable cholesterol-lowering method. Volixibat is an apical sodium-dependent bile acid transporter inhibitor that blocks the reabsorption of bile acids, causing the liver to produce more bile acids, lowering cholesterol, and also improving insulin sensitivity. A phase IIa clinical trial of volixibat is currently enrolling patients with NASH, with a primary endpoint of improvement in NAFLD Activity Score without worsening of fibrosis.[59]

GS-9674 is a nonsteroidal FXR agonist with encouraging results from phase I study. These data demonstrated the biological activity and safety profile of this agent, which is being tested further in NASH phase IIa clinical trials.

Agents Targeting Lipid Metabolism

Fenofibrates, as discussed, are not the only medication group that alters the lipid metabolism. In fact, it has been known for a long time that NAFLD is accompanied by a dyslipidemic metabolic state in most patients and statins have been used for the treatment of hyperlipidemia in patients with NAFLD.[62] Also, the literature shows that the risk for serious liver injury from statins is rare and patients with NAFLD and hyperlipidemia are not at an increased risk for statin hepatotoxicity.[62] However, statins have antiinflammatory, antioxidant, and antithrombotic effects that are independent of their lipid-lowering activity. In this context, statins have been proposed for the treatment of NAFLD and NASH.[63] Although simvastatin, rosuvastatin, and pitavastatin can be used successfully to treat hyperlipidemia in patients with NAFLD, none of these agents have been shown to improve histology or reduce liver-related morbidity and mortality.[63]

In contrast, aramchol is a synthetic lipid molecule, obtained by conjugating 2 natural compounds, namely, cholic acid, which is a bile acid, and arachidic acid, which is a saturated fatty acid. It is an SCD-1 inhibitor, which is the enzyme that catalyzes the rate-limiting step in monounsaturated fatty acid synthesis. A randomized, double-blind, placebo-controlled study by Safadi and colleagues[64] showed that aramchol was safe and effective in reducing liver fat content, as measured by magnetic resonance spectroscopy after 12 weeks of daily administration of 300 mg.

Another way to decrease hepatic triglyceride levels is the use of thyroid hormone receptor β agonists. It was previously shown that NAFLD and NASH are associated with liver-specific hypothyroidism, caused by decreased thyroid hormone–regulated gene expression in the liver.[65] Moreover, hypothyroidism is associated with increased triglyceride and cholesterol levels. It has been proposed that thyroid hormone receptor β agonists, by their action in the liver, can decrease triglyceride levels and increase reverse cholesterol metabolism. MGL-3196 is an example of thyroid hormone receptor β agonists and a phase IIa trial is currently enrolling patients with NASH to investigate the hepatic fat change caused by MGL-3196.[59]

Finally, another agent that affects lipid metabolism is GS-0976, which is an acetyl coenzyme A (CoA) carboxylase inhibitor. In this way, it inhibits the conversion of acetyl CoA to malonyl CoA, and ultimately functions to downregulate steatosis. GS-0976 is being assessed in a phase IIa clinical trial for its effect on patients with NASH. There is also a combination agent, GS-0976 + GS-9674, which is the grouping of an acetyl CoA carboxylase inhibitor and an FXR agonist, and is underway for a phase IIa clinical trial for its safety and tolerability in patients with NASH.

Other Agents Currently Under Investigation

JKB-121, which is nalmefene, is an opioid receptor antagonist and works through Toll-like receptor 4 antagonism. This receptor is present in Kupffer and stellate cells, as well as in hepatocytes. It has been used in alcohol dependence and pruritus in cholestasis before. Currently, JKB-121 is being studied in a phase IIa clinical trial, for its effects on NASH.

SUMMARY

NAFLD is a very common metabolic condition with an increasing prevalence around the world, for which various treatment strategies have been developed. NAFLD is not always benign; it has been shown in myriad studies that NASH can lead to advanced liver disease. In clinic, lifestyle modification has been the initial approach for the management of NAFLD, although it is not sustainable in the majority of cases. Pharmacologic agents have been emerging for the treatment of NAFLD, targeting 1 or more steps in the NAFLD pathogenesis. A great deal of effort has been focused on the treatment of NASH with significant fibrosis, to develop safe and effective therapeutic regimens.

REFERENCES

1. Sayiner M, Koenig A, Henry L, et al. Epidemiology of nonalcoholic fatty liver disease and nonalcoholic steatohepatitis in the United States and the rest of the world. Clin Liver Dis 2016;20(2):205–14.
2. Golabi P, Sayiner M, Fazel Y, et al. Current complications and challenges in nonalcoholic steatohepatitis screening and diagnosis. Expert Rev Gastroenterol Hepatol 2016;10(1):63–71.

3. Younossi ZM, Koenig AB, Abdelatif D, et al. Global epidemiology of nonalcoholic fatty liver disease-Meta-analytic assessment of prevalence, incidence, and outcomes. Hepatology 2016;64(1):73–84.

4. Fazel Y, Koenig AB, Sayiner M, et al. Epidemiology and natural history of nonalcoholic fatty liver disease. Metabolism 2016;65(8):1017–25.

5. Canbay A, Sowa JP, Syn WK, et al. NASH Cirrhosis - the new burden in liver transplantation: how should it be managed? Visc Med 2016;32(4):234–8.

6. Younossi ZM, Stepanova M, Negro F, et al. Nonalcoholic fatty liver disease in lean individuals in the United States. Medicine (Baltimore) 2012;91(6):319–27.

7. Kumar R, Rastogi A, Sharma MK, et al. Clinicopathological characteristics and metabolic profiles of non-alcoholic fatty liver disease in Indian patients with normal body mass index: do they differ from obese or overweight non-alcoholic fatty liver disease? Indian J Endocrinol Metab 2013;17(4):665–71.

8. Younossi ZM, Blissett D, Blissett R, et al. The economic and clinical burden of nonalcoholic fatty liver disease in the United States and Europe. Hepatology 2016;64(5):1577–86.

9. Golabi P, Otgonsuren M, Cable R, et al. Non-alcoholic fatty liver disease (NAFLD) is associated with impairment of health related quality of life (HRQOL). Health Qual Life Outcomes 2016;14:18.

10. Bazick J, Donithan M, Neuschwander-Tetri BA, et al. Clinical model for NASH and advanced fibrosis in adult patients with diabetes and NAFLD: guidelines for referral in NAFLD. Diabetes Care 2015;38(7):1347–55.

11. Noureddin M, Anstee QM, Loomba R. Review article: emerging anti-fibrotic therapies in the treatment of non-alcoholic steatohepatitis. Aliment Pharmacol Ther 2016;43(11):1109–23.

12. Fabbrini E, Mohammed BS, Magkos F, et al. Alterations in adipose tissue and hepatic lipid kinetics in obese men and women with nonalcoholic fatty liver disease. Gastroenterology 2008;134(2):424–31.

13. Tilg H, Moschen AR. Evolution of inflammation in nonalcoholic fatty liver disease: the multiple parallel hits hypothesis. Hepatology 2010;52(5):1836–46.

14. Buzzetti E, Pinzani M, Tsochatzis EA. The multiple-hit pathogenesis of non-alcoholic fatty liver disease (NAFLD). Metabolism 2016;65(8):1038–48.

15. Chalasani N, Younossi Z, Lavine JE, et al. The diagnosis and management of non-alcoholic fatty liver disease: practice guideline by the American Gastroenterological association, American association for the study of liver diseases, and American College of Gastroenterology. Gastroenterology 2012;142(7):1592–609.

16. Sofi F, Macchi C, Abbate R, et al. Mediterranean diet and health. Biofactors 2013; 39(4):335–42.

17. Ryan MC, Itsiopoulos C, Thodis T, et al. The Mediterranean diet improves hepatic steatosis and insulin sensitivity in individuals with non-alcoholic fatty liver disease. J Hepatol 2013;59(1):138–43.

18. Sofi F, Casini A. Mediterranean diet and non-alcoholic fatty liver disease: new therapeutic option around the corner? World J Gastroenterol 2014;20(23): 7339–46.

19. Promrat K, Kleiner DE, Niemeier HM, et al. Randomized controlled trial testing the effects of weight loss on nonalcoholic steatohepatitis. Hepatology 2010;51(1): 121–9.

20. Luyckx FH, Desaive C, Thiry A, et al. Liver abnormalities in severely obese subjects: effect of drastic weight loss after gastroplasty. Int J Obes Relat Metab Disord 1998;22(3):222–6.

21. Johnson NA, Keating SE, George J. Exercise and the liver: implications for therapy in fatty liver disorders. Semin Liver Dis 2012;32(1):65–79.

22. Golabi P, Locklear CT, Austin P, et al. Effectiveness of exercise in hepatic fat mobilization in non-alcoholic fatty liver disease: systematic review. World J Gastroenterol 2016;22(27):6318–27.

23. Burton GW, Joyce A, Ingold KU. Is vitamin E the only lipid-soluble, chain-breaking antioxidant in human blood plasma and erythrocyte membranes? Arch Biochem Biophys 1983;221(1):281–90.

24. Pacana T, Sanyal AJ. Vitamin E and nonalcoholic fatty liver disease. Curr Opin Clin Nutr Metab Care 2012;15(6):641–8.

25. Sanyal AJ, Chalasani N, Kowdley KV, et al. Pioglitazone, vitamin E, or placebo for nonalcoholic steatohepatitis. N Engl J Med 2010;362(18):1675–85.

26. Lavine JE, Schwimmer JB, Van Natta ML, et al. Effect of vitamin E or metformin for treatment of nonalcoholic fatty liver disease in children and adolescents: the TONIC randomized controlled trial. JAMA 2011;305(16):1659–68.

27. Stampfer MJ, Rimm EB. Epidemiologic evidence for vitamin E in prevention of cardiovascular disease. Am J Clin Nutr 1995;62(6 Suppl):1365S–9S.

28. Rimm EB, Stampfer MJ, Ascherio A, et al. Vitamin E consumption and the risk of coronary heart disease in men. N Engl J Med 1993;328(20):1450–6.

29. Syn WK, Choi SS, Diehl AM. Apoptosis and cytokines in non-alcoholic steatohepatitis. Clin Liver Dis 2009;13(4):565–80.

30. Zein CO, Yerian LM, Gogate P, et al. Pentoxifylline improves nonalcoholic steatohepatitis: a randomized placebo-controlled trial. Hepatology 2011;54(5):1610–9.

31. Du J, Ma YY, Yu CH, et al. Effects of pentoxifylline on nonalcoholic fatty liver disease: a meta-analysis. World J Gastroenterol 2014;20(2):569–77.

32. Nati M, Haddad D, Birkenfeld AL, et al. The role of immune cells in metabolism-related liver inflammation and development of non-alcoholic steatohepatitis (NASH). Rev Endocr Metab Disord 2016;17(1):29–39.

33. Lefebvre E, Moyle G, Reshef R, et al. Antifibrotic effects of the dual CCR2/CCR5 antagonist cenicriviroc in animal models of liver and kidney fibrosis. PLoS One 2016;11(6):e0158156.

34. Friedman S, Sanyal A, Goodman Z, et al. Efficacy and safety study of cenicriviroc for the treatment of non-alcoholic steatohepatitis in adult subjects with liver fibrosis: CENTAUR phase 2b study design. Contemp Clin Trials 2016;47:356–65.

35. Sanyal AJ, Harrison S, Abdelmalek MF, et al. Cenicriviroc vs Placebo for treatment of nonalcoholic steatohepatitis with fibrosis: results from the year 1 primary analysis of the phase 2b CENTUAR study. Hepatology 2016;64:1118A–9A.

36. Tobira. AURORA: Phase 3 Study for the Efficacy and Safety of CVC for the Treatment of Liver Fibrosis in Adults With NASH. 2017. Available at: https://clinicaltrials.gov/ct2/show/NCT03028740. Accessed April 2, 2017.

37. Loomba R, Lawitz E, Mantry P, et al. GS-4997, an inhibitor of apoptosis signal-regulating kinase (ASK1), Alone or in combination with simtuzumab for the treatment of nonalcoholic steatohepatitis (NASH): a randomized, phase 2 trial. Hepatology 2016;64:1119A–20A.

38. Adar T, Ben Ya'acov A, Lalazar G, et al. Oral administration of immunoglobulin G-enhanced colostrum alleviates insulin resistance and liver injury and is associated with alterations in natural killer T cells. Clin Exp Immunol 2012;167(2):252–60.

39. Grygiel-Gorniak B. Peroxisome proliferator-activated receptors and their ligands: nutritional and clinical implications–a review. Nutr J 2014;13:17.

40. Neuschwander-Tetri BA, Brunt EM, Wehmeier KR, et al. Improved nonalcoholic steatohepatitis after 48 weeks of treatment with the PPAR-gamma ligand rosiglitazone. Hepatology 2003;38(4):1008–17.
41. He L, Liu X, Wang L, et al. Thiazolidinediones for nonalcoholic steatohepatitis: a meta-analysis of randomized clinical trials. Medicine (Baltimore) 2016;95(42): e4947.
42. Pai V, Paneerselvam A, Mukhopadhyay S, et al. A multicenter, prospective, randomized, double-blind study to evaluate the safety and efficacy of saroglitazar 2 and 4 mg Compared to Pioglitazone 45 mg in Diabetic Dyslipidemia (PRESS V). J Diabetes Sci Technol 2014;8(1):132–41.
43. Fukunaga T, Zou W, Rohatgi N, et al. An insulin-sensitizing thiazolidinedione, which minimally activates PPARgamma, does not cause bone loss. J Bone Miner Res 2015;30(3):481–8.
44. Tyagi S, Gupta P, Saini AS, et al. The peroxisome proliferator-activated receptor: a family of nuclear receptors role in various diseases. J Adv Pharm Technol Res 2011;2(4):236–40.
45. Ratziu V, Harrison SA, Francque S, et al. Elafibranor, an agonist of the peroxisome proliferator-activated receptor-alpha and -delta, induces resolution of nonalcoholic steatohepatitis without fibrosis worsening. Gastroenterology 2016;150(5): 1147–59.e5.
46. Ruzehaji N, Frantz C, Ponsoye M, et al. Pan PPAR agonist IVA337 is effective in prevention and treatment of experimental skin fibrosis. Ann Rheum Dis 2016; 75(12):2175–83.
47. Joshi SR. Saroglitazar for the treatment of dyslipidemia in diabetic patients. Expert Opin Pharmacother 2015;16(4):597–606.
48. Doycheva I, Loomba R. Effect of metformin on ballooning degeneration in nonalcoholic steatohepatitis (NASH): when to use metformin in nonalcoholic fatty liver disease (NAFLD). Adv Ther 2014;31(1):30–43.
49. Nauck M. Incretin therapies: highlighting common features and differences in the modes of action of glucagon-like peptide-1 receptor agonists and dipeptidyl peptidase-4 inhibitors. Diabetes Obes Metab 2016;18(3):203–16.
50. Kim W, Egan JM. The role of incretins in glucose homeostasis and diabetes treatment. Pharmacol Rev 2008;60(4):470–512.
51. Oseini AM, Sanyal AJ. Therapies in non-alcoholic steatohepatitis (NASH). Liver Int 2016;37(Suppl 1):97–103.
52. Carbone LJ, Angus PW, Yeomans ND. Incretin-based therapies for the treatment of non-alcoholic fatty liver disease: a systematic review and meta-analysis. J Gastroenterol Hepatol 2016;31(1):23–31.
53. Armstrong MJ, Barton D, Gaunt P, et al. Liraglutide efficacy and action in nonalcoholic steatohepatitis (LEAN): study protocol for a phase II multicentre, double-blinded, randomised, controlled trial. BMJ Open 2013;3(11):e003995.
54. Kenny PR, Brady DE, Torres DM, et al. Exenatide in the treatment of diabetic patients with non-alcoholic steatohepatitis: a case series. Am J Gastroenterol 2010; 105(12):2707–9.
55. Ohki T, Isogawa A, Toda N, et al. Effectiveness of ipragliflozin, a sodium-glucose co-transporter 2 inhibitor, as a second-line treatment for non-alcoholic fatty liver disease patients with type 2 diabetes mellitus who do not respond to incretin-based therapies including glucagon-like peptide-1 analogs and dipeptidyl peptidase-4 inhibitors. Clin Drug Inves 2016;36(4):313–9.
56. Neuschwander-Tetri BA, Loomba R, Sanyal AJ, et al. Farnesoid X nuclear receptor ligand obeticholic acid for non-cirrhotic, non-alcoholic steatohepatitis (FLINT):

a multicentre, randomised, placebo-controlled trial. Lancet 2014;385(9972): 956–65.

57. Brodosi L, Marchignoli F, Petroni ML, et al. NASH: a glance at the landscape of pharmacological treatment. Ann Hepatol 2016;15(5):673–81.

58. Miyata M, Sakaida Y, Matsuzawa H, et al. Fibroblast growth factor 19 treatment ameliorates disruption of hepatic lipid metabolism in farnesoid X receptor (Fxr)-null mice. Biol Pharm Bull 2011;34(12):1885–9.

59. Harrison S. Emerging Trends in Non-alcoholic Fatty Liver Disease-Emerging therapies for NASH: Non-antifibrotics. 2017. Available at: http://liverlearning.aasld. org/aasld/2017/emerging_trends_conference/169509/stephen.harrison.emerging. therapy.for.nash.non-antifibrotics.html?f=p6m1e1169c10698. Accessed April 7, 2017.

60. Liu J, Xu Y, Hu Y, et al. The role of fibroblast growth factor 21 in the pathogenesis of non-alcoholic fatty liver disease and implications for therapy. Metabolism 2014; 64(3):380–90.

61. Hussainzada N, Banerjee A, Swaan PW. Transmembrane domain VII of the human apical sodium-dependent bile acid transporter ASBT (SLC10A2) lines the substrate translocation pathway. Mol Pharmacol 2006;70(5):1565–74.

62. Abel T, Feher J, Dinya E, et al. Safety and efficacy of combined ezetimibe/simvastatin treatment and simvastatin monotherapy in patients with non-alcoholic fatty liver disease. Med Sci Monit 2009;15(12). MS6-11.

63. Pastori D, Polimeni L, Baratta F, et al. The efficacy and safety of statins for the treatment of non-alcoholic fatty liver disease. Dig Liver Dis 2014;47(1):4–11.

64. Safadi R, Konikoff FM, Mahamid M, et al. The fatty acid-bile acid conjugate Aramchol reduces liver fat content in patients with nonalcoholic fatty liver disease. Clin Gastroenterol Hepatol 2014;12(12):2085–91.e1.

65. Eshraghian A, Hamidian Jahromi A. Non-alcoholic fatty liver disease and thyroid dysfunction: a systematic review. World J Gastroenterol 2014;20(25):8102–9.

Wilson Disease
Diagnosis, Treatment, and Follow-up

Michael L. Schilsky, MD

KEYWORDS

- Wilson disease • Copper • Ceruloplasmin • Liver failure

KEY POINTS

- Consideration of a diagnosis of Wilson disease is still the critical factor in testing for and establishing disease diagnosis.
- In association with other clinical and biochemical tests, liver biopsy results and molecular genetic testing can be used to generate a score for diagnosing Wilson disease.
- Medical therapy is effective for most patients; liver transplant can rescue those with acute liver failure or those with advanced liver disease who fail to respond to or discontinue medical therapy.
- Treatment monitoring must be done at regular intervals and includes clinical evaluation, liver tests and blood counts, and copper metabolic parameters.

INTRODUCTION

Sir Samuel Alexander Kinnier Wilson, the American born and British-trained neurologist for whom this disorder is named, was the first who linked the occurrence of the neurologic degenerative disease with cirrhosis of the liver that was mostly identified at autopsy in his patients. It is now more than a century since the publication of his landmark thesis[1] and there is now a clear understanding of the disease pathophysiology and its underlying genetic defect. This knowledge has led to earlier clinical recognition of disease and improvement in diagnostics useful for generating clinical algorithms and scoring systems to aid clinicians. The focus of this review is to aid practicing gastroenterologists in identify patients with Wilson disease in a timely fashion and allow them to initiate appropriate therapy and treatment monitoring.

Disclosure: Dr. M.L. Schilsky is an investigator for WTX101 trial (Wilson therapeutics, sponsor), advisor for GMPO and Kadmon, serves on the Chair medical advisory committee for the Wilson Disease Association.
Yale University Medical Center, 333 Cedar Street, LMP 1080, New Haven CT 06520, USA
E-mail address: Michael.Schilsky@Yale.edu

Clin Liver Dis 21 (2017) 755–767
http://dx.doi.org/10.1016/j.cld.2017.06.011
1089-3261/17/© 2017 Elsevier Inc. All rights reserved.

liver.theclinics.com

PATHOGENESIS AND EPIDEMIOLOGY

The underpinning mechanism of Wilson disease is a defect in ATP7B, a copper transporting ATPase that is mainly expressed in hepatocytes.[2] This altered function is due to mutation of the *ATP7B* gene, for which there are more than 500 known disease-associated mutations at present. Therefore, in North America, where there is no single dominant mutation, most patients are compound heterozygotes with a different mutation on each allele of the gene that is localized to chromosome 13.[3] The disease is thought to be 100% penetrant but with variable phenotype.

The incidence of Wilson disease is commonly quoted as approximately 1:30,000; however, more recent genetic studies from the United Kingdom question whether there is a higher gene frequency.[4] There are some unique populations where there is an increased disease incidence thought to be related to consanguinity, and here there are often dominant mutations of *ATP7B*.[5,6]

In Wilson disease patients with absent or dysfunctional ATP7B, the normal biliary copper excretion required for copper homeostasis is reduced and copper accumulates in liver cells. This accumulation of copper eventually overwhelms safe storage capacity and cellular injury occurs.[2] The degree of liver disease and timing for its expression is variable in individuals, making this a challenging diagnosis in some patients. The variability is likely due to differences in dietary intake of copper, the natural source for this essential element, and an individual's antioxidant capacity, susceptibility to hepatic fibrosis, and hormonal influences. Evidence for the extragenic influences on disease expression comes from siblings with the same genetic defect that express widely variable phenotypes.[7] In addition, patients may have other hepatic disorders in concert with Wilson disease, and this may accelerate disease progression.[8]

When the liver's capacity for copper storage is exceeded, and when liver cells are injured, copper is released into the circulation and may accumulate in other organs, notably the central nervous system, where it may cause neurologic and psychiatric disease as well as give rise to the characteristic Kayser-Fleischer corneal deposits of copper. Most Wilson disease patients typically present with liver disease during their first and second decades of life. By contrast, patients with neurologic or psychiatric symptoms and disease present in the second and third decades or later on.[9] There are exceptions, however, and patients have been diagnosed with Wilson disease in their eighth decade of life with severe or mild symptoms.[10]

The low level of circulating ceruloplasmin found in most patients with Wilson disease is directly related to defective copper handling in hepatocytes as a result of mutation of *ATP7B*. ATP7B functions in biliary copper excretion but also in moving copper into the trans-Golgi network, the biosynthetic compartment, where the peptide of ceruloplasmin acquires its complement of copper and reaches its final folded state before release into the circulation.[11] Without the normal complement of copper, the peptide folds differently and its circulating half-life is reduced,[12] leading to the phenotypic finding of a low level of ceruloplasmin in the circulation of patients with Wilson disease. A lack of ceruloplasmin by itself does not lead to copper accumulation, as shown by the rare disorder aceruloplasminemia. This disorder results from a defect in the ceruloplasmin gene with a failure of ceruloplasmin synthesis by liver cells, but there is no hepatic copper accumulation, rather iron-induced neurodegeneration.[13,14]

DIAGNOSIS OF WILSON DISEASE

Wilson disease can be diagnosed with increased accuracy given better understanding of the disorder and also the addition of molecular diagnostic testing. Over the years since Wilson made the diagnosis by the recognition of the neurologic findings in his patients, the ability to recognize specific phenotypic markers of disease and test with liver tests and liver biopsy and other biochemical testing for ceruloplasmin and copper has vastly improved diagnostic capabilities. One thing that has not changed with time, however, is that if the diagnosis of Wilson disease is not sought, there can be delays or a failure to make the diagnosis at all. Therefore, to help in establishing a diagnosis, clinicians must be alert as to when to consider Wilson disease. Discussed later and in **Table 1** are scenarios for when to consider a diagnosis of Wilson disease. In addition, when Wilson disease is considered in the differential diagnosis, it is important to know when the diagnostic evaluation is completed to establish a diagnosis or if further evaluation is still needed to exclude this disorder.

In an attempt to help clinicians better understand how to evaluate patients for Wilson disease, a gathering of experts in Leipzig, Germany, helped establish a weighted diagnostic scoring system using clinical, biochemical, and, for the first time, molecular genetic testing for Wilson disease.[15] This has come to be known as the Leipzig criteria, and its use has been validated in adult and pediatric populations and incorporated into guidelines put forth by the European Association for the Study of the Liver.[16] Using this scoring system, a clinician may tabulate results from individual tests, and, if the score is 4 or above, the diagnosis is established.

The only difficulty with the Leipzig criteria scoring system is that when used in isolation it does not give clinicians an algorithmic approach as to which testing order should be considered first. In general, I favor noninvasive testing first. Therefore, along with an ophthalmologic examination, blood and urine testing and nowadays molecular testing should be performed first. Liver biopsy is typically performed when these are not diagnostic or to evaluate the degree of hepatic inflammation and for hepatic copper quantitation. When the time comes where testing for mutations of the Wilson disease gene, *ATP7B*, becomes inexpensive and rapid, this test may be a starting point for diagnostic testing. At present, cost and logistics sometimes limit the use of the molecular testing, but these barriers are likely to change with time. The approach to some unique clinical scenarios where Wilson disease must be differentiated from patients with other liver disease is discussed.

DIAGNOSIS—CLINICAL SCENARIOS
The Patient with Unexplained Liver Disease

Perhaps the most common scenario warranting consideration for a diagnosis of Wilson disease for the gastroenterologist is patients with unexplained liver disease or abnormal liver tests (**Box 1**). Most commonly, history helps in excluding alcoholic liver disease or drug-induced liver injury; however, there may be overlap with other disorders both in the presence of hepatic inflammation and some serologic markers of autoimmune liver disease or viral hepatitis. In answering when it is proper to test for Wilson disease, before or after or simultaneous with testing for other liver diseases, the first question to ask patients is whether there is a family history of early neurologic, psychiatric, or unexplained liver disease or if they themselves have neurologic or psychiatric disease. Neurologic disease most often presents with tremor and progresses with gait imbalance, dysarthria, drooling, and at times severe symptoms that mimic parkinsonism. Psychiatric disease may range widely from a mild mood disturbance to frank psychosis, but most often there is some element of depression.

If the answer is yes to any of these signs or symptoms, then testing for Wilson disease should proceed. Similarly, if a liver biopsy is performed for diagnostic purposes without the initial consideration for Wilson disease, then histologic findings of glycogenated nuclei and steatosis (micro or macro) should prompt further testing for Wilson disease and the remaining liver core used for quantitation of copper.

Table 1 Leipzig scoring system	
Typical clinical symptoms and signs	
KF rings	
Present	2
Absent	0
Neurologic symptoms[b]	
Severe	2
Mild	1
Absent	0
Testing	
Serum ceruloplasmin	
Normal (>0.2 g/L)	0
0.1–0.2 g/L	1
<0.1 g/L	2
Coombs-negative hemolytic anemia	
Present	1
Absent	0
Other tests	
Liver copper (in the absence of cholestasis)	
>5 × ULN (>4 μmol/g)	2
0.8–4 μmol/g	1
Normal (<0.8 μmol/g)	−1
Rhodanine-positive granules[a]	1
Urinary copper (in the absence of acute hepatitis)	
Normal	0
1–2 × ULN	1
>2 × ULN	2
Normal, but >5 × ULN after D-penicillamine	2
Mutation analysis	
On both chromosomes +	4
On 1 chromosome +	1
No mutations +	0
Total score evaluation	
4 or more diagnoses established	
3 diagnoses possible, more tests needed	
2 or fewer diagnoses very unlikely	

Abbreviation: ULN, upper limit of normal.
  [a] If no quantitative liver copper available.
  [b] Or typical abnormalities at brain magnetic resonance imaging.
  From Ferenci P, Caca K, Loudianos G, et al. Diagnosis and phenotypic classification of Wilson disease. Liver Int 2003;23(3):141; with permission.

Other scenarios where Wilson disease should be sought and where a patient likely has some liver abnormality include those with the presence of Fanconi syndrome, low levels of serum uric acid, and presence or history of nonimmune hemolytic anemia. Rare fortuitous detection of Kayser-Fleischer (KF) rings on ophthalmologic

---

Box 1
When to test for Wilson disease

Test early for Wilson disease if there is liver disease and any of the following
- A family history of neurologic or psychiatric disease with early onset
- A family history of unexplained and progressive liver disease
- A history of neurologic or psychiatric signs or symptoms
- A low level of serum uric acid
- Fanconi syndrome
- Histologic changes on liver biopsy consistent with Wilson disease
- Steatosis/steatohepatitis on a biopsy in which nonalcoholic fatty liver disease is unexpected

---

examination or brain MRI findings suggestive of Wilson disease (changes in basal ganglia or pons most commonly), even without clear liver disease, should prompt a search for Wilson disease. When these nonhepatic findings are present in concert with liver disease, there is an increased probability of Wilson disease being present.

Therefore, if any of these are present, then the testing for Wilson disease needs to be exhaustive. Patients should have a formal ophthalmologic slit-lamp examination for KF rings, but those presenting with liver disease without neuropsychiatric symptoms may have these present only approximately 50% of the time, and the absence of findings should not suspend further evaluation. Serum testing should be conducted for ceruloplasmin, urine 24-hour collection performed for copper, and a liver biopsy with copper quantitation should be considered. With the advent of noninvasive testing for fibrosis and molecular testing for *ATP7B* mutations, liver biopsy may be needed less often because the diagnosis and staging of liver disease can often be established without these. There are less frequent patients identified with negative testing for *ATP7B* mutations given the improved molecular testing now available; however, the absence of mutations gives reason for the performance of a liver biopsy and copper quantitation to help establish diagnosis of the liver disease.

The Patient with a Low Ceruloplasmin

Testing for serum ceruloplasmin is often performed as part of the battery of testing in looking for the cause of unexplained liver disease. The degree of change in the serum level of ceruloplasmin connotes differences in the predictive value of the finding for establishing a diagnosis of Wilson disease[17]; however, there are several instances when the value may be lower than normal and a patient does not have Wilson disease (**Box 2**). One of the most common scenarios is the presence of a carrier state for Wilson disease because 20% of carriers have a nonpathologic lower than normal level of this serum protein. When considering an isolated value of a low serum ceruloplasmin, it is, therefore, approximately 40 times more common to see carriers with low ceruloplasmin than patients. When there are other findings, however, as discussed previously, that increase the suspicion for Wilson disease, the predictive value likely rises.

The recognition of copper deficiency is something that has arisen due to the neurologic presentation of individuals postoperatively with altered absorption or in those patients chronically exposed to increased dietary zinc.[18,19] Copper deficiency can lead to neurologic symptoms more akin to other disorders affecting the posterior columns of the spinal tracts than the typical changes seen in Wilson disease. In these individuals, serum copper is very low in proportion to the lower serum ceruloplasmin level, and urine copper is also low. This differs from most symptomatic Wilson disease patients where the low ceruloplasmin is accompanied by an increased amount of circulating copper not bound to ceruloplasmin and also an increased urine copper

---

Box 2
Reasons for a low level of serum ceruloplasmin

- Wilson disease
- Carrier (heterozygote) for Wilson disease
- Copper deficiency
- Nephropathy with loss of large proteins in the urine
- Enteropathy with loss of proteins in the gut
- Excess zinc ingestion
- Menkes disease or other *ATP7A* mutations
- Aceruloplasminemia or carrier state for this disorder

---

excretion. There can be hepatic histologic changes with steatosis in some patients with copper deficiency (Dr P. Ferenci, MD, personal communication, 2017) and in animal models of copper deficiency.[20]

There are other rarer scenarios where the serum copper and ceruloplasmin may be low. In Menkes disease and in variants of this disorder where cellular copper transport is affected by mutations in *ATP7A*, copper absorption is impaired and copper and ceruloplasmin levels may be low.[21] Other clinical signs and symptoms of this disorder predominate (neurodegenerative changes early in life and skeletal abnormalities for those later with milder disease) and copper levels do not accumulate significantly in the liver or other sites. Another rare disorder of the ceruloplasmin gene, aceruloplasminemia, results in absence of ceruloplasmin in the circulation and, in carriers, approximately 50% of the amount of ceruloplasmin normally seen. This disorder is sometimes accompanied by iron overload and neurologic injury later in life.[14]

The Patient with Acute Liver Failure

Approximately 5% of patients with Wilson disease present with acute liver failure.[22] These patients are typically in their second or third decade of life, have an associated nonimmune hemolytic anemia, and, for the purposes of diagnosis, characteristically altered ratios of alkaline phosphatase to bilirubin (<1:4) and aspartate aminotransferase to alanine aminotransferase (>2.2) that allow the identification of these individuals even before confirmatory copper studies or molecular testing is available. Often there seems to be some precipitating event, a flu-like illness or some possible drug reaction, but not always. These patients almost invariably progress with liver failure rapidly with increased jaundice, exacerbated by the hemolysis, ascites, and hepatic encephalopathy. All these patients have underlying fibrosis or cirrhosis that went undetected until their critical presentation. These patients should be evaluated for liver transplantation as soon as possible given the almost invariable progression to further liver failure and death.[22,23] Rare instances of rescue with medical therapy have been reported; however, most of these patients are advanced at the time of their presentation, and many have associated renal injury and even hepatorenal syndrome that makes initiation of medication that requires renal excretion, D-penicillamine or trientine, less useful.

The proportion of patients who develop acute liver failure due to Wilson disease who are female has increased. It is probable that hormonal influences are responsible for their increased susceptibility based on studies in an animal model of Wilson disease, the Long-Evans Cinnamon rat. When female Long-Evans Cinnamon rats are subject to ovarectomy, there is a slight delay their presentation with severe liver injury and a higher mortality during this part of their disease.[24] Other investigators have speculated an autoimmune phenomenon after initial injury with exposure to cryptic antigens as another mechanism for accelerated liver injury that occurs in an animal models for Wilson disease.[25]

In patients with known Wilson disease who stop treatment, the same development of acute liver failure has been reported. The interval from the time of stoppage of therapy to the development of liver failure is variable, but there are reports of this taking 1 year to 2 years.[26] In some patients, however, who were either nonadherent to a low copper diet or to their medical treatment prior to its total stoppage, the time to progression is sooner. It is difficult to give an exact time for this to occur due to patient dietary differences, differences in length of treatment, type of treatment, and adherence to treatment, as discussed previously.

Family Screening After Disease Diagnosis

Once an individual is identified with Wilson disease, it is mandatory that siblings be tested as well. Testing is best performed by molecular diagnosis if a patient's mutations can be identified. There are some patients, however, with only a single mutation and less commonly no mutation identified at all who require standard testing, as discussed previously, to further explore the diagnosis of Wilson disease. Urine copper should not be using in isolation for screening siblings because it can be normal in asymptomatic patients.

Other first-degree relatives of patients should be tested for Wilson disease. In young patients who are diagnosed with Wilson disease, I recommend testing parents. Offspring also should be tested. Both parents and offspring need to be tested by standard clinical and biochemical testing because a parent or child is at minimum an obligate heterozygote and has 1 copy of the gene inherited from the patient but the other copy inherited from the other parent or grandparent.

TREATMENT AND MONITORING OF WILSON DISEASE

Once a diagnosis of Wilson disease is established, treatment must be initiated. There are treatments necessary related to Wilson disease and also adjunctive therapies that apply to all or only some patients. The latter include low copper diet, management of complications of portal hypertension, and management of neurologic and psychiatric symptoms.

Treatment of Wilson Disease

In Roberts and my guidelines for the American Association for the Study of Liver Diseases,[9] medical therapy is divided into 2 categories: treatment of symptomatic patients and treatment of asymptomatic patients. The rationale for this separation arises from the presumption that in symptomatic patients, disease progression is likely more rapid and arresting, and reversing the copper-related injury is more time sensitive. In asymptomatic patients, the goal instead is prevention of the development of symptoms, and this may be accomplished with less urgency. After some time of initial treatment, symptomatic patients then become stable or asymptomatic, and treatment is then considered maintenance therapy. It is fortunate that for those failing medical therapy or with acute liver failure, liver transplantation for Wilson disease can be performed with results showing excellent survival.[27] Guidance for choosing transplantation or continued treatment with medical therapy can use objective data derived from the testing of patients (discussed later).

Medical Therapy—Symptomatic Patients

Treatment of symptomatic patients (hepatic, neurologic, or psychiatric) should include chelation therapy, either with ᴅ-penicillamine or with trientine that increases urinary copper excretion. The dosages of both are given from 2 times to 4 times daily, titrated up to an approximate weight-based dosing of approximately 20 mg/kg body weight for initial therapy. The duration of time for initial treatment dosing is not strictly defined, but it is thought that this represents a decoppering period of treatment, where copper is removed from the mobile more toxic pools of cellular copper. After liver tests and hepatic synthetic function have improved, typically in 6 months' to 12 months' time, the treatment dosage may be reduced to a maintenance therapy using a dose of approximately 10-15 mg/kg body weight of ᴅ-penicillamine or trientine. An alternative for this transition to maintenance therapy with lower-dose chelation is the use of zinc salts to prevent copper absorption from the gut. Zinc is typically given as 50 mg of elemental zinc in a zinc salt (eg, zinc acetate, zinc sulfate, zinc gluconate, and other forms) in adults, dosed 3 times daily.

All these medications for Wilson disease are typically given apart from food, either 1 hour before or 2 hours after meals. Administration with food inhibits the absorption and effectiveness of the medication.

Goals of therapy for patients with liver disease are initially disease stabilization and then reversal of injury and improvement in liver function in those with impaired function at the outset. Failures of therapy include those with symptom and biochemical progression despite treatment, and, in these individuals, liver transplantation may need to be considered as rescue therapy. To aid in deciding if medical therapy or transplantation is needed, a modified King's Wilson disease score can be calculated for patients[28] (**Table 2**). Elements for this score include bilirubin, international normalized ratio (INR), and albumin along with the white blood cell count. Although there are individual exceptions, a score of 10 or more suggests that liver transplantation is most likely to be needed, whereas those with scores of less than 10 most often can be treated medically. A lowering of the modified King's Wilson score with treatment in a patient at or approaching a score of 10 suggests reassessment of the need for considering liver transplant; likewise, an increasing score despite treatment should accelerate a transplant evaluation and listing for transplant.

Medical Therapy—Asymptomatic Patients

Treatment of asymptomatic patients aims to prevent disease progression and development of symptoms. Therefore, recommended treatment of asymptomatic patients

Table 2
Modified King's Wilson disease score

	1[a]	2[a]	3[a]	4[a]
Serum bilirubin (μmol/L)	100–150	151–200	201–300	>300
AST (U/L)	100–150	151–300	301–400	>400
INR	1.3–1.6	1.7–1.9	2.0–2.4	>2.4
White blood cell count (10⁹/L)	6.8–8.3	8.4–10.3	10.4–15.3	>15.3
Albumin (g/L)	34–44	25–33	21–24	<21

[a] Score points, upper limit of normal for AST = 20 IU/mL (at King's College). A score ≥11 is associated with high probability of death without liver transplantation.

Data from Nazer H, Ede RJ, Mowat AP, et al. Wilson's disease: clinical presentation and use of prognostic index. Gut 1986;27:1377–81; and Dhawan A, Taylor RM, Cheeseman P, et al. Wilson's disease in children: 37-year experience and revised King's score for liver transplantation. Liver Transplant 2005;11:441–8.

includes either chelation, D-penicillamine, or trientine, given at a reduced dosage of 10 mg/kg to 15 mg/kg in 2 to 4 divided dosages, or zinc salts, given as 50 mg 3 times daily for adults and 25 mg 3 times daily for pediatric patients. Treatment choice can be tailored to a patient's needs and tolerance of medication, but unless patients experience a side effect of therapy, they are likely to be able to choose whichever treatment they and their treating physician feel comfortable and have experience with.

Special Considerations and Medication Intolerance

Treatment choices and dosing of medication may need to take into account a patient's future needs, such as pregnancy in younger women, and other needs, such as wound healing or planned surgical procedures. For pregnancy, chelator dosages should be reduced by 50% at time of conception and maintained at this level during the pregnancy with monitoring performed during each trimester. Zinc therapy may be continued uninterrupted during pregnancy.[29] With respect to surgical procedures, there is a concern that chelation can remove copper from proteins, such as lysyl oxidase that crosslinks collagen, and, therefore, in patients with wounds or planned surgery, a lower dosage of chelation (approximately 50% reduction) is used; alternatively, patients may take zinc therapy.

Medication intolerance becomes an issue for a minority of patients on medical therapy but may result in a change in therapy in 25% to 30% of treated patients.[30] Patients treated with D-penicillamine may be subject to several side effects, early and late, that may necessitate change of medication. Early reactions include hypersensitivity and nephritis and a lupus-like syndrome and marrow toxicity as well as infrequent increase in liver tests. Later reactions include dermatologic changes and nephrotic syndrome and rare myasthenia. The frequency of drug reaction to trientine is far less, but some patients experience gastric dyspepsia and rarely colitis, although this has been reported for D-penicillamine as well.[31] The main issue with zinc treatment is gastric dyspepsia, occurring in approximately 20% of those on zinc therapy. This may be in part be related to the salt coupled with the zinc, and sometimes patients need to alter their zinc preparation. Other concerns regarding zinc are the slightly higher failure rate for control hepatic disease,[30] but whether some of these patients who did poorly in this study were failures due to nonadherence or to other medical complications, such as secondary liver disease, is uncertain.

Adjunctive Treatment of Wilson Disease

Patients with Wilson disease are counseled to eat a diet low in copper and avoid the very high copper foods, such as mushrooms, chocolate, liver, and nuts. Whether addition of vitamin supplements to aid antioxidant defenses is efficacious or not is uncertain, but data from animal studies of copper overload suggested addition of vitamin E might be useful for reducing oxidative injury. Avoidance of other injurious medications and herbal compounds is recommended for Wilson disease as it is for other liver disease patients, along with immunization for preventable viral hepatitis A and B in nonimmune patients.

If patients have cirrhosis and portal hypertension or have clinical evidence or other surrogates, such as thrombocytopenia, to suggest they might, they should have screening for esophageal and gastric varices and undergo primary prophylaxis with β-blockers if present. For those with esophageal varices and nontolerance of β-blockers, banding of varices can be performed. Screening and surveillance for hepatocellular carcinoma may be performed when cirrhosis is present, but whether the threshold for the incidence of this complication is above the 2.5% incidence recommended for screening and surveillance and merits actual formal recommendations for its routine performance in Wilson disease is uncertain.

Monitoring

Monitoring of treatment is for treatment efficacy, adherence to treatment, and side effects of therapy. After treatment initiation of symptomatic patients, clinical and biochemical monitoring should be more intensive and tailored to a patient's degree of illness and potential for clinical worsening. For example, a patient with a high modified King's Wilson score, typically 7 or above, with decompensated cirrhosis or unstable neurologic symptoms may be seen or monitored weekly or twice monthly, while the dosage of medication is increased to goal and then less frequently once there is disease stability.

After this initiation of treatment, during the initial year of therapy, patients should be seen every 3 months and then afterward at 6-month intervals. This period for monitoring helps detect those with difficulty with or nonadherence to therapy. Adherent patients should demonstrate normalization of liver tests in the vast majority with time, typically over the first 6 months to 18 months of treatment.

Some liver tests in patients with advanced liver disease may not reach normal values but should stabilize during this same interval and may still slowly improve with time. Examples of improvement over time are increase in serum albumin, decrease in INR, and increase in platelet counts. Whether these reach normal values or not may depend on the degree of impairment and portal hypertension at the outset, response and adherence to therapy and diet, and whether there are any secondary reasons for liver injury.

Testing to be monitored at visits is outlined in **Box 3**. Testing should follow blood counts with platelets to monitor for medication side effects and overtreatment, the latter associated with the development of anemia, neutropenia, and thrombocytopenia from a relative copper deficiency at critical blood cell production sites. Liver tests help define if there is improvement or prevention of inflammation, and albumin and INR the synthetic function of the liver. Urinalysis is to monitor for nephritis and proteinuria.

Monitoring of copper status is important for helping adjust medication dosing as well as responding to treatment failure and nonadherence to therapy. In most symptomatic patients basal urine copper excretion is elevated above 100 μg daily, and with the initiation of chelation therapy this is typically increased 10-fold or more. Over time this is reduced to approximately 150 μg to 250 μg daily in patients on trientine, and 250 μg to 500 μg those on D-penicillamine treatment. By contrast, for patients on zinc with elevated initial urine copper, the urine excretion decreases with treatment. In **Table 3**, treatment goals for urine copper excretion for each treatment are discussed.

Box 3
Tests for monitoring patients with Wilson disease

- Complete blood cell count and platelets
- Liver panel — alanine aminotransferase, aspartate aminotransferase, alkaline phosphatase, total and direct bilirubin
- Copper testing — serum copper, serum ceruloplasmin
- Urinalysis (for those on D-penicillamine and trientine)
- 24-hour urine for copper
- 24-hour urine for zinc (in zinc treated patients)

Treatment	Treatment Goal	Undertreatment or Nonadherence	Overtreatment or Nonadherence
D-Penicillamine	250–500	>500	<150
Trientine	150–250	>500	<100
Zinc	30–120	>120	<30

Table 3
Urine copper excretion on treatment of Wilson disease

Another way to follow copper status is to simultaneously determine total serum copper (micrograms per deciliter) and subtract ceruloplasmin copper (ceruloplasmin in milligrams per deciliter times 3.15) to calculate the nonceruloplasmin or free copper. Most well treated patients typically have values between 5 µg/dL and 15 µg/dL. Unfortunately, using commonly commercially available immunologic methods for determination of ceruloplasmin values, the calculation of nonceruloplasmin copper may be low or even negative in 20% of patients, and, in these patients, other parameters, clinical examination, liver tests, and urine copper may be used in concert to manage adjustment of therapy.

Monitoring of adherence includes history and clinical examination, testing for liver enzymes, and estimate of nonceruloplasmin copper and urine copper excretion. In addition, for patients on zinc, excretion of zinc in the urine indicates adherence to treatment and helps confirm good absorption.

New Treatment Innovation

Currently available treatments are typically given in multiple daily dosages apart from food to insure absorption. This often leads to nonadherence in missed dosages or dosages with less than optimal efficacy if taken with food. A pilot study was conducted with 8 patients using once a fixed weight–based once-daily dosing of trientine (20 mg/kg body weight) for Wilson disease to determine if this was adequate therapy.[32] After 1 year of treatment, patients did well without any stoppages of treatment due to worsening disease. Urine copper excretion remained within therapeutic goals for these patients on treatment. Patient survey indicated that the once-daily dosing improved adherence to medication and was more desirable to patients. A larger clinical study is needed to show safety and establish dose ranging for once-daily treatment with currently available chelators for Wilson disease.

Previous studies with sodium tetrathiomolybdate for the treatment of Wilson disease suggested some benefit for its use as initial treatment of patients with neurologic Wilson disease.[33] A recent phase 2 study was conducted of a more stable form of a chelator for copper, choline tetrathiomolybdate (WTX101), that has the potential to increase biliary copper excretion as well as bind copper and albumin in an inert complex in the circulation; 28 patients with Wilson disease were enrolled, 89% with neurologic Wilson disease, most treated for less than 90 days but all treated for less than 2 years. All patients had reductions in circulating nonceruloplasmin copper by 8 weeks to 12 weeks and improvement in neurologic status in all who completed the 24 weeks of therapy. Although there were liver enzyme elevations in approximately one-third of patients, these were reversible with dose reduction or treatment holiday and were not associated with increased bilirubin. Importantly, no early (within 12 weeks) neurologic deterioration was seen during the early phase of treatment. Further testing of this compound is warranted to determine its role in the future armamentarium for the treatment of Wilson disease.[34]

SUMMARY

Consideration of a diagnosis of Wilson disease is still the critical factor in testing for and establishing disease diagnosis. In association with other clinical and biochemical tests, liver biopsy results and molecular genetic testing can be used to generate a score for diagnosing Wilson disease. Medical therapy is effective therapy for most patients; liver transplant can be used to rescue those with acute liver failure or those with liver disease who fail to respond to medical therapy. Treatment monitoring must be done at regular intervals and includes clinical evaluation, liver tests and blood counts, and copper metabolic parameters. Outcomes with medical therapy or transplantation are excellent for most patients with Wilson disease. New advances in treatment may improve adherence and reduce some complications of treatment.

REFERENCES

1. Wilson SAK. Progressive lenticular degeneration: a familial nervous disease associated with cirrhosis of the liver. Brain 1912;34:295–507.
2. Schilsky ML, Thiele D. Copper metabolism and the liver. In: Arias IM, Wolkoff AE, Boyer JL, et al, editors. The liver: biology and pathobiology. 5th Edition. Chichester (UK): John Wiley & Sons, Ltd; 2009. p. 221–33.
3. Bennett J, Hahn SH. Clinical molecular diagnosis of Wilson disease. Semin Liver Dis 2011;31:233–8.
4. Coffey AJ, Durkie M, Hague S, et al. A genetic study of Wilson's disease in the United Kingdom. Brain 2013;136:1476–87.
5. Gialluisi A, Incollu S, Pippucci T, et al. The homozygosity index (HI) approach reveals high allele frequency for Wilson disease in the Sardinian population. Eur J Hum Genet 2013;21:1308–11.
6. García-Villarreal L, Daniels S, Shaw SH, et al. High prevalence of the very rare Wilson disease gene mutation Leu708Pro in the Island of Gran Canaria (Canary Islands, Spain): a genetic and clinical study. Hepatology 2000;32:1329–36.
7. Ala A, Schilsky ML. Genetic modifiers of liver injury in hereditary liver disease. Semin Liver Dis Ed P Burk 2011;31:208–14.
8. Wong RJ, Gish R, Schilsky M, et al. A clinical assessment of Wilson disease in patients with concurrent liver disease. J Clin Gastroenterol 2011;45(3):267–73.
9. Roberts E, Schilsky ML. A practice guideline on Wilson disease. Hepatology 2008;47:2089–111.
10. Ala A, Borjigin J, Rochwarger A, et al. Wilson disease in septuagenarian siblings: raising the bar for diagnosis. Hepatology 2005;41:668–70.
11. Terada K, Nakako T, Yang XL, et al. Restoration of holoceruloplasmin synthesis in LEC rat after infusion of recombinant adenovirus bearing WND cDNA. J Biol Chem 1998;273(3):1815–20.
12. Holtzman NA, Gaumnitz BM. Studies on the rate of release and turnover of ceruloplasmin and apoceruloplasmin in rat plasma. J Biol Chem 1970;245:2354–8.
13. Edwards CQ, Williams DM, Cartwright GE. Hereditary hypoceruloplasminemia. Clin Genet 1979;15:311–6.
14. Xu X, Pin S, Gathinji M, et al. Aceruloplasminemia: an inherited neurodegenerative disease with impairment of iron homeostasis. Ann N Y Acad Sci 2004;1012: 299–305.
15. Ferenci P, Caca K, Loudianos G, et al. Diagnosis and phenotypic classification of Wilson disease. Liver Int 2003;23(3):139–42.
16. Ferenci P, Czlonkowska A, Stremmel W, et al. EASL clinical practice guidelines: Wilson's disease. European association for study of liver. J Hepatol 2012;56:671–85.

17. Mak CM, Lam CW, Tam S. Diagnostic accuracy of serum ceruloplasmin in Wilson disease: determination of sensitivity and specificity by ROC curve analysis among ATP7B-genotyped subjects. Clin Chem 2008;54:1356–62.

18. Kumar N, Gross JB Jr, Ahlskog JE. Myelopathy due to copper deficiency. Neurology 2003;61:273–4.

19. Jaiser SR, Winston GP. Copper deficiency myelopathy. J Neurol 2010;257: 869–81.

20. Medici V. The evolving scenario of copper and fatty liver. Metab Syndr Relat Disord 2013;11:4–6.

21. Kaler SG. ATP7A-related copper transport disorders. In: Pagon RA, Adam MP, Ardinger HH, et al, editors. GeneReviews® [Internet]. Seattle (WA): University of Washington, Seattle; 2003. p. 1993–2017. Available at: https://www.ncbi.nlm.nih.gov/books/NBK1413/. Accessed July 31, 2017.

22. Reuben A, Tillman H, Fontana RJ, et al. Improved outcomes in adults with acute liver failure (ALF) from 1998 to 2013: an update from the US Acute Liver Failure Study Group. Ann Intern Med 2016;164:724–32.

23. Sokol RJ, Francis PD, Gold SH, et al. Orthotopic liver transplantation for acute fulminant Wilson disease. J Pediatr 1985;107:549–52.

24. Kasai N, Miyoshi I, Osanai T, et al. Effects of sex hormones on fulminant hepatitis in LEC rats: a model of Wilson's disease. Lab Anim Sci 1992;42:363–8.

25. Yokoi T, Nagayama S, Kajiwara R, et al. Identification of protein disulfide isomerase and calreticulin as autoimmune antigens in LEC strain of rats. Biochim Biophys Acta 1993;1158:339–44.

26. Herbert Scheinberg IH, Jaffe ME, Sternlieb I. The use of trientine in preventing the effects of interrupting penicillamine therapy in Wilson's Disease. N Engl J Med 1987;317:209–13.

27. Arnon R, Annunziato R, Schilsky M, et al. Liver transplantation for children with Wilson disease: comparison of outcomes between children and adults. Clin Transplant 2011;25:E52–60.

28. Dhawan A, Taylor RM, Cheeseman P, et al. Wilson's disease in children: 37-Year experience and revised King's score for liver transplantation. Liver Transpl 2005; 11:441–8.

29. Brewer GJ, Johnson VD, Dick RD, et al. Treatment of Wilson's disease with zinc. XVII: treatment during pregnancy. Hepatology 2000;31:364–70.

30. Weiss KH, Thurik F, Gotthardt DN, et al, EUROWILSON Consortium. Efficacy and safety of oral chelators in treatment of patients with Wilson disease. Clin Gastroenterol Hepatol 2013;11:1028–35.

31. Boga S, Jain D, Schilsky ML. Trientine induced colitis during therapy for Wilson disease: a case report and review of the literature. BMC Pharmacol Toxicol 2015;16:30.

32. Ala A, Aliu E, Schilsky ML. Once daily trientene for maintenance therapy for Wilson disease. Dig Dis Sci 2015;60:1433–9.

33. Brewer GJ, Askari F, Lorincz MT, et al. Treatment of Wilson disease with ammonium tetrathiomolybdate: IV. Comparison of tetrathiomolybdate and trientine in a double-blind study of treatment of the neurologic presentation of Wilson disease. Arch Neurol 2006;63:521–7.

34. Heinz WK, Aftab A, Frederick A, et al. WTX101 in patients newly diagnosed with Wilson disease: final results of a global, prospective phase 2 trial. Amsterdam: EASL; 2017. Late Breaking Abstract.

Acute Liver Failure

Chalermrat Bunchorntavakul, MD[a,b], K. Rajender Reddy, MD[b,*]

KEYWORDS

- Acute liver failure • Cerebral edema • Encephalopathy • *N*-acetylcysteine
- Liver transplantation • Extracorporeal liver support system • Liver dialysis

KEY POINTS

- Acute liver failure is a life-threatening condition of heterogeneous etiology.
- Outcomes are better with early recognition and prompt initiation of etiology-specific therapy, complex intensive care protocols, and urgent liver transplantation.
- Cerebral edema and intracranial hypertension (ICH) are reasons for high morbidity and mortality.
- Hypertonic saline is suggested for patients with high-risk for developing ICH and, when ICH develops, mannitol is recommended as a first-line therapy.

INTRODUCTION

Acute liver failure (ALF) is a rare but life-threatening condition. The most widely accepted definition includes the evidence of hepatic necrosis, coagulation abnormality (International Normalized Ratio $\geq$1.5), and any degree of mental alteration (encephalopathy) in a patient without preexisting cirrhosis and with a duration of illness of less than 26 weeks. Patients with Wilson disease, perinatally acquired hepatitis B virus (HBV), or autoimmune hepatitis may be included, despite the presence of underlying cirrhosis, if their disease has only been recognized for less than 26 weeks. It is important to appreciate that ALF is a distinct entity from an acute exacerbation of chronic liver disease (or acute-on-chronic liver failure). For instance, acute alcoholic hepatitis is not considered to be ALF. ALF can be further classified based on the time interval between the development of jaundice and encephalopathy[1–4] (**Table 1**). It should be noted that the onset of encephalopathy is often sudden, may precede jaundice, asterixis may be transient, and, unlike chronic liver disease, may be associated with agitation, changes in personality, delusions, and restlessness.[5]

Conflict of Interest: The authors have nothing to disclose.
[a] Division of Gastroenterology and Hepatology, Department of Medicine, Rajavithi Hospital, College of Medicine, Rangsit University, Rajavithi Road, Ratchathewi, Bangkok 10400, Thailand; [b] Division of Gastroenterology and Hepatology, Department of Medicine, Hospital of the University of Pennsylvania, University of Pennsylvania, 2 Dulles, 3400 Spruce Street, Philadelphia, PA 19104, USA
* Corresponding author.
E-mail address: rajender.reddy@uphs.upenn.edu

Clin Liver Dis 21 (2017) 769–792
http://dx.doi.org/10.1016/j.cld.2017.06.002
1089-3261/17/© 2017 Elsevier Inc. All rights reserved.

Table 1
Classification of acute liver failure

	Interval Between Onset of Encephalopathy from Jaundice	Common Etiologies	Clinical Presentation	Prognosis
Hyperacute	<7 d	APAP, HAV, ischemic	Cerebral edema common	Fair (survival without LT ~36%)
Acute	7–21 d	HBV, drugs	Cerebral edema less common	Poor (survival without LT ~14%)
Subacute	22 d to <26 wk	drugs, indeterminate	Cerebral edema rare; ascites, peripheral edema and renal failure more common	Very poor (survival without LT ~7%)

Abbreviations: APAP, acetaminophen; HAV, hepatitis A virus; HBV, hepatitis B virus; LT, liver transplantation.

Over the last 3 decades, ALF has evolved from a poorly understood condition with a near entirely fatal outcome, to one with a relatively well-characterized phenotype and disease course.[6,7] Complex intensive care protocols and urgent liver transplantation (LT), as well as specific therapy according to the etiology, have been used promptly as a standard of care for ALF. Accordingly, the overall and LT-free survival rates of patients with ALF have been improving through the past few decades and the majority of patients may now be expected to survive, particularly where LT is available.[6,8]

ETIOLOGY

The etiology of ALF varies greatly by country and also has changed over time.[9–11] Over the past few decades, the most common etiology of ALF has evolved, with hepatitis A and B on the decline in incidence, while acetaminophen (APAP) and other medications related ALF have been on the increase, at least in the United States and Western Europe.[6,9–11] In the United States and the UK, APAP overdose currently accounts for 45% to 60% of cases of ALF, with viral hepatitis and idiosyncratic drug reactions each accounting for 10% to 12% of cases.[6,9–11] Notably, the incidence of APAP overdose also varies among developed countries, because it accounts for only 3% to 9% of ALF in Spain and Germany, reflecting the differences in behavior and perhaps in the national regulatory system with regard to access to large doses of APAP.[12,13] By contrast, Asia Pacific countries have a higher incidence of ALF owing to hepatitis viruses, specifically hepatitis E virus in India and Pakistan, and HBV in Japan, Hong Kong, Thailand, as well as Australia, with fewer cases of APAP overdose being observed.[6,10,11,14]

Common and uncommon etiologies of ALF are listed in **Table 2**. Apart from the well-known causes of drug-induced ALF, several recently introduced agents (eg, tyrosine kinase inhibitors, monoclonal antibodies, dabigatran, rivaroxaban, lamotrigine, levetiracetam, pregabalin, venlafaxine, duloxetine, sertraline, darunavir, and maraviroc) and herbal supplements (eg, black cohosh, germander, chaparral, kava kava, Chinese herbs, and anthraquinones) have also been reported to cause ALF.[15,16] Important clinical characteristics, prognosis, and specific therapies of selected etiologies of ALF, including viruses,[17–24] medications,[25–27] autoimmune,[28,29] Wilson disease,[30]

Table 2
Etiology of acute liver failure

Infections	Viral hepatitis A, B, C, D, E
	Herpes simplex virus, varicella zoster virus
	Epstein-Barr virus, cytomegalovirus
	Tropical infections (eg, Dengue virus, leptospirosis, scrub typhus, malaria)
Drug and toxins	Acetaminophen
	Carbon tetrachloride
	Idiosyncratic drug reactions (eg, modern medications,[a] herbal supplements)
	Mushroom poisoning (eg, *Amanita phalloides*)
	Sea anemone sting
Ischemia	Ischemic hepatitis, hypoperfusion, cardiogenic shock
	Heat stroke
	Cocaine, methamphetamines, ephedrine, ecstasy
Vascular	Acute Budd-Chiari syndrome
	Sinusoidal obstruction syndrome
Miscellaneous	Autoimmune hepatitis
	Wilson disease
	Reye syndrome
	Malignant infiltration
	Acute fatty liver of pregnancy, eclampsia, HELLP syndrome
	Primary graft nonfunction after liver transplantation
	Indeterminate

Abbreviation: HELLP, hemolysis, elevated liver enzymes, low platelets.

[a] Isoniazid, rifampicin, pyrazinamide, sulfonamides, trimethoprim-sulfamethoxazole, amoxicillin-clavulanate, dapsone, ketoconazole, ofloxacin, didanosine, efavirenz, allopurinol, diclofenac, halothane, isoflurane, phenytoin, valproic acid, nicotinic acid, statins, imipramine, propylthiouracil, disulfiram, lisinopril, labetalol, methyldopa, amiodarone, flutamide, metformin, etoposide, gemtuzumab.

mushrooms,[31–34] ischemia,[35] and Budd-Chiari syndrome,[36] are summarized in **Table 3**.[3,5,10,11] Indeterminate etiology, despite extensive workup, continues to be a sizable ALF group (12%–43% of cases), even in the Western world.[4,6,12]

DIAGNOSIS

A thorough medical history should be obtained and physical examination should be done promptly. A history of potential exposures to viral infections, drugs, herbs, and other toxins should be explored. If encephalopathy is present, the history may be unavailable or can only be provided by the family. Early testing should include routine chemistries, arterial blood gas, complete blood counts, blood typing, APAP level, screening for other drugs and toxins, viral serologies, tests for Wilson disease, autoantibodies, and a pregnancy test in females. Thus, testing for complications such as acute pancreatitis should also be performed[3,4] (**Box 1**).

APAP–protein adducts are released into blood during hepatocyte lysis and the concentration of adducts in the serum has been noted to correlate with the degree of APAP hepatotoxicity. Thus, it may be a rapid and useful diagnostic test for ALF of unknown cause or unclear history, and for patients who present more than 1 day after APAP overdose.[25,37,38] Interestingly, up to 19% of indeterminate cases in the US Acute Liver Failure Study Group (US-ALFSG) study demonstrated adducts in serum suggesting that unrecognized APAP toxicity caused or contributed to ALF in these patients.[39] Liver biopsy, most often done via the transjugular route, is generally not recommended in the setting of ALF.[40,41] It is indicated only when certain conditions such

Table 3
Clinical characteristics, prognosis and specific therapy of selected etiologies of ALF

Etiologies	Clinical Characteristics	Prognosis of ALF	Specific Therapy
Hepatitis A	• Lives in or traveled to endemic area • Ingestion of contaminated food and water, particularly shellfish • ALF develops in ~0.35% of acute hepatitis A (more common in older patients and those with preexisting liver disease)	• Mortality ~40% without LT	• Not available
Hepatitis B	• Lives in or traveled to endemic area • Known or unknown HBV, recovered HBV infection and exposed to immunosuppressant, B-cell–depleting agents, and cancer chemotherapy • ALF develops in 0.4%–4% of acute hepatitis B	• Mortality >60%–80% without LT (higher mortality if reactivated by immunosuppressive therapy, B-cell–depleting agents, and cancer chemotherapy)	• Nucleos(t)ide analogues (preferably entecavir or tenofovir)
Hepatitis E	• Lives in or traveled to endemic area • Ingestion of contaminated water in endemic areas • ALF develops in 0.2%–0.5% of acute hepatitis E (increased dramatically to 15%–25% in pregnant women, particularly in the third trimester)	• Mortality 45% without LT (better prognosis compared with other etiologies of ALF in India)	• Not available
APAP	• Ingestion of APAP >7.5–10 g (4–10 g in high-risk population; eg, alcoholics, cirrhotics, taking CYP2E1 inducers) • Marked elevation of ALT (often >3000 IU/L and AST > ALT), starts increasing 24–36 h after overdose • Relatively low level of bilirubin • Early metabolic acidosis and elevated lactate • ARF (10%–50%) and pancreatitis (0.3%–5%) may develop	• More favorable outcomes compared with other causes of ALF, but it still has a high mortality (~30%) • Low phosphate may be seen as a good prognostic maker (but replacement is required)	• NAC IV: 150 mg/kg load, then 12.5 mg/kg/h × 4 h, then 6.25 mg/kg/h • Activate charcoal if presented within 4 h after ingestion

Cause	Clinical features	Prognosis	Treatment
Non-APAP DILI	• Exposures to certain medications or herbs (in the United States, the most common implicated agents were antimicrobials) • More often in older patients • Latent period typically 4 d to 8 wk • Hypersensitivity reactions may be present in more than one-third of patients • May have subacute clinical course mimicking cirrhosis	• Mortality ~70% without LT • CAM-induced ALF is associated with higher rates of LT and lower LT-free survival compared with prescription medicine	• Discontinuation of suspicious agent(s) • Corticosteroids may be of benefit in selected patients with hypersensitivity reactions
Autoimmune hepatitis	• Often subacute presentation • Young or middle-age women • High serum gamma-globulins • Positive serum autoantibodies	• Mortality >50% without LT	• Prednisolone 40–60 mg/d and discontinue in 7–10 d if no improvement (in the context of ALF, steroids are often ineffective and may favor septic complications)
Wilson disease	• Child or young adults • Coombs-negative hemolytic anemia • Rapid progression to renal failure • Relative mild rises in ALT (often AST > ALT) • Normal or subnormal ALP (typically <40 IU/L) • TB (mg/dL)/ALP (IU/L) ratio >2	• Usually fatal without LT	• LT must be promptly considered • Albumin dialysis, hemofiltration or plasmapheresis may lower serum copper and limit further hemolysis • D-Penicillamine is not recommended in ALF
Mushroom poisoning	• Ingestion of wild mushroom, mainly Amanita phalloides, A verna, A virosa • Preceded by muscarinic effects, such as profuse sweating, vomiting and diarrhea within 6–12 h after ingestion, then clinical hepatotoxicity often develops after 24-48 h	• Mortality 30%–60% without LT • LT should be strongly considered if interval between ingestion and diarrhea <8 h, PT index[a] <10% or PT index <25% + Cr ≥1.2 mg/dL from d 3–4 after ingestion	• Penicillin G: 1 g/kg/d IV • Silibinin 5 mg/kg IV q4h • NAC (as for APAP)
Herpes simplex virus	• Immunocompromised host and pregnant women (but can also occur in normal host) • Classic triad: high fever, leukopenia, marked elevation of ALT • Mucocutaneous vesicles present in ~50%	• 74% progressed to death or LT (51% in acyclovir-treated patients and 88% in untreated patients)	• Acyclovir: 5–10 mg/kg IV q8h

(continued on next page)

Table 3
(continued)

Etiologies	Clinical Characteristics	Prognosis of ALF	Specific Therapy
Epstein-Barr virus	• Young adults • 25% immunosuppressed • Classical symptoms of infectious mononucleosis may not be present • 50% have cholestatic injury	• Mortality 50%–75% without LT	• Antiviral agents (eg, acyclovir, ganciclovir, famciclovir) • Corticosteroids
Ischemic hepatitis	• Associated with cardiac or pulmonary disease (~30% of patients) • Cardiopulmonary precipitant was identified in 70% • Marked elevation of ALT (>1000 IU/L; AST > ALT), increased LDH and Cr; with normalization soon after stabilization of hemodynamic instability	• Mortality ~ 30% without LT • Higher serum phosphate and grade 3 or 4 encephalopathy are associated with poor outcomes	• Optimizing hemodynamic status and cardiopulmonary conditions
Budd-Chiari syndrome	• 84% female • 63% have hypercoagulable state • Abdominal pain, hepatomegaly, ascites • AST/ALT ratio >1 • Diagnosis: Doppler ultrasound imaging (loss of hepatic venous signal of reverse flow in PV), computed tomography, MRI	• Mortality 50%–60% even with the availability of LT • Higher peak ALT and Cr are associated with poorer outcomes	• Early anticoagulation followed by TIPS and/or LT
Malignant infiltration	• Common malignancies are lymphoma, leukemia, breast and colon cancer • History of cancer (75% for breast cancer, but only 10% for lymphoma or leukemia) • Massive hepatomegaly • Elevated ALP and/or other tumor markers • About 50% have liver mass on imaging • Liver biopsy may be required for diagnosis	• Near 100% mortality (90% died within 3 wk)	• Chemotherapy

Abbreviations: ALF, acute liver failure; ALP, alkaline phosphatase; ALT, alanine aminotransferase; APAP, acetaminophen; ARF, acute renal failure; AST, aspartate aminotransferase; CAM, complementary and alternative medicines; Cr, creatinine; DILI, drug-induced liver injury; HBV, hepatitis B virus; IV, intravenous; LDH, lactate dehydrogenase; LT, liver transplantation; NAC, N-acetylcysteine; PV, portal veins; TIPS, transjugular intrahepatic portosystemic shunt.

[a] PT index; prothrombin time control plasma/prothrombin time patient plasma] × 100.

Box 1
Initial laboratory tests in patients with acute liver failure

- Chemistries: sodium, potassium, chloride, bicarbonate, calcium, magnesium, phosphate, glucose, aspartate aminotransferase, alanine aminotransferase, alkaline phosphatase, gamma glutamyl transferase, total bilirubin, albumin, creatinine, blood urea nitrogen, lactate dehydrogenase, creatinine kinase

- Urine output (hourly)

- Complete blood count, blood type and screen

- Prothrombin time, International Normalized Ratio, fibrinogen

- Arterial blood gas

- Arterial lactate

- Ammonia (arterial if possible)

- Acetaminophen level, toxicology screen

- Viral hepatitis serologies: anti-hepatitis A virus IgM, hepatitis B surface antigen, anti-hepatitis B core antigen IgM, anti-hepatitis E virus,[d] anti-hepatitis C virus, hepatitis C virus RNA[a], herpes simplex virus-1 IgM, varicella zoster virus

- Ceruloplasmin level[b]

- Pregnancy test (females)

- Autoimmune markers: antinuclear antibody, anti-smooth muscle antibody, anti-soluble liver antigen, anti-neutrophil cytoplasmic antibody, immunoglobulin levels

- Human immunodeficiency virus-1, human immunodeficiency virus-2[c]

- Amylase and lipase

- Tests for tropical infections[d]

[a] Done to recognize potential underlying infection.
[b] Done only if Wilson disease is a consideration (eg, in patients <40 years without another obvious explanation for acute liver failure [ALF]); in this case, the uric acid level and bilirubin to alkaline phosphatase ratio and serum copper may be helpful as well. Ceruloplasmin may be falsely low in non-Wilson ALF owing to massive hepatic necrosis or may be increased owing to it being an acute phase reactant. Because Wilson disease has a low prevalence in the ALF population, there is a great likelihood that any test for Wilson disease would have a high negative predictive value but a low positive predictive value.
[c] Implications for potential liver transplantation.
[d] If clinically indicated.
Data from Lee WM, Stravitz, Larson AM. AASLD position paper: the management of acute liver failure: update 2011. The American Association for the Study of Liver Diseases. Available at: https://www.aasld.org/sites/default/files/guideline_documents/alfenhanced.pdf and European Association for the Study of the Liver. J Hepatol 2017;66(5):1047–81.

---

as autoimmune hepatitis, metastatic liver disease, lymphoma, or herpes simplex virus are suspected.[3] Liver histology also could predict the outcomes in ALF, because greater than 50% hepatocyte necrosis is associated with a 3-fold higher mortality.[40,41] Liver imaging studies may disclose malignant infiltrations or Budd-Chiari syndrome, but are seldom definitive.

PROGNOSTIC FACTORS AND SCORING SYSTEM

It is well-known that ALF is a severe and life-threatening condition, and the chance of spontaneous recovery is variable according to the presentation and etiology. A number of factors influence survival of patients and one of the most important predictors of outcome is the etiology of ALF: LT-free survival is greater than 50% for ALF associated with APAP, hepatitis A, ischemia, and pregnancy, compared with less than 25% for other causes.[5,42] In addition, the severity of encephalopathy also impacts survival significantly (spontaneous recovery: 65%–70% with grade 1 or 2, 40%–50% with grade 3, and <20% with grade 4 encephalopathy).[5,43] Those who survive rarely develop cirrhosis. Two-year outcomes in initial survivors are generally good, but non-APAP patients have a significantly lower survival (75.5% compared with 89.5% in APAP overdose survivors, which may be related to preexisting medical comorbidities.[44] In contrast, spontaneous survivors with APAP overdose experience substantial morbidity during follow-up from ongoing psychiatric and substance abuse issues.[44]

LT is the only life-saving procedure for some patients with ALF. Identifying the right patient for LT in a timely manner is vital and therefore several prognostic scoring systems have been developed. The Kings College Criteria (KCC) was the first validated scoring system (introduced in 1989) and is currently the most widely used prognostic tool for ALF (**Table 4**). It has good specificity (82%–94%), but has limited sensitivity (68%–82%).[5,43,45,46] The positive predictive values are reasonable (70%–90%), but negative predictive values are variable (25%–90%). Therefore, a significant number of patients who do not fulfill the KKC will eventually die without LT.[5,43,45,46] In addition, the KCC performs best in groups with high-grade encephalopathy and in historically earlier studies suggesting that modern medical management of ALF may modify performance of KCC because its sensitivity was reduced in studies published after 2005 (46%–71%) compared with studies before 1995 (76%–82%).[46] Arterial blood lactate greater than 3.5 mmol/L is an early predictor of mortality in APAP-associated ALF (sensitivity 67%, specificity 95%, positive predictive value 79%, negative predictive value 91%) and may increase the predictive accuracy of the KCC.[47]

Other prognostic systems for ALF have been proposed including the Model for End-stage Liver Disease (MELD) score,[48] Clichy criteria,[49–51] and Acute Physiology and Chronic Health Evaluation II score.[52] In a systematic analysis of the MELD score in ALF, 526 patients with ALF from 6 studies (all did not have LT support, which may not be a good representation of the Western populations) were included and overall

Table 4 King's College criteria	

Acute liver failure owing to acetaminophen	• Arterial pH <7.3 or lactate >3 mmol/L after adequate fluid resuscitation and >24 h since ingestion
	• All 3 following criteria:
	  ○ Grade III or IV encephalopathy
	  ○ Serum creatinine >3.4 mg/dL (>300 μmol/L)
	  ○ INR >6.5 (PT >100 s)

Acute liver failure not owing to acetaminophen	• INR >6.5 (PT >100 s)
	• 3 out of 5 following criteria:
	  ○ Unfavorable etiology: indeterminate, Wilson disease, idiosyncratic drug reaction
	  ○ Age <10 y or >40 y
	  ○ Jaundice for >7 d before development of encephalopathy
	  ○ Bilirubin >17 mg/dL (>300 μmol/L)
	  ○ INR >3.5 (PT >50 s)

Abbreviations: INR, International Normalized Ratio; PT, prothrombin time.

304 died (58%). By using a MELD score cutoff of 30.5 to 35, the pooled sensitivity was 77% (95% CI, 72%–82%) and specificity was 72% (95% CI, 62%–80%). The positive likelihood ratio was 2.76 (95% CI, 1.97–3.87) and negative likelihood ratio was 0.31 (95% CI, 0.25–0.40).[41] The differences between KKC and MELD are slight, although it seems that the KCC is more specific and the MELD score is more sensitive.[40,41] Accordingly, the American Gastroenterological Associates suggests using the MELD score rather than the KCC as a prognostic scoring system in patients presenting with ALF (a cutoff MELD score of 30.5 should be used for prognosis and higher scores predict a need for LT).[40] A more recent European Association for the Study of the Liver guideline recommends that LT be considered in those patients fulfilling either the KCC or Clichy criteria.[4] A factor V level of less than 20% may indicate a poor prognosis necessitating consideration of LT in patients of 30 years of age or younger, and a higher threshold of less than 30% is of equivalent significance in older patients.[49–51] Recently, by using data from the US-ALFSG, a logistic regression model to predict LT-free survival has been developed using admission variables include hepatic encephalopathy (HE) grade, ALF etiology, vasopressor use, bilirubin, and International Normalized Ratio.[53] In the validation cohort, this model was noted to be superior to KCC and MELD, with a c-statistic value of 0.84, 66.3% accuracy, 32.5% sensitivity, and 95.3% specificity; however, external validations are required.[53]

Apart from these scoring systems, other serum laboratory parameters (eg, alfa-fetoprotein,[54] Gc-globulin,[55] phosphate,[56] galectin-9,[57] procoagulant microparticles,[58] soluble CD163,[59] and liver-type fatty acid binding protein[60]) and etiology-specific prognostic systems (eg, hepatitis A virus,[20] idiosyncratic drug reaction,[61,62] Wilson disease,[30] autoimmune hepatitis,[29] and *Amanita phalloides* poisoning[31,32]) for predicting outcomes in ALF have also been proposed.[10]

MANAGEMENT

ALF is considered a "hepatology emergency" in that early discussion with a transplant team and/or rapid transfer to an experienced center that has LT availability is advisable once a patient is stabilized. Acute onset of jaundice and elevated transaminases and prolonged International Normalized Ratio, but without encephalopathy, is acute liver injury and not ALF. Most patients with APAP-associated acute liver injury recover, whereas patients with non–APAP-associated acute liver injury more readily may evolve on to ALF.[63] Levels of alanine aminotransferase do not necessarily correlate with the severity of liver injury and do not have to be markedly elevated in ALF (particularly in ALF related to acute fatty liver of pregnancy and Wilson disease), and International Normalized Ratio, bilirubin, and severity of HE are the key indicators of clinical severity.[4] Certain etiologies of ALF may require specific therapies promptly (see **Table 3**). Given the severity and rarity of the disease, most of these interventions have not been evaluated in a well-designed study, and the use of them is often based on the basis of pathogenesis, studies in animals, or in patients without ALF. Therefore, the true benefit of these interventions in patients with ALF is unclear, recognizing that patients with ALF can spontaneously recover.

Because ALF often leads to infections and multiple organ failures, admission to the intensive care unit should be considered as early as possible, especially when HE and/or coagulopathy is progressing. Careful monitoring and general management to prevent and treat infections and the use of organ support systems, where applicable and available, are very important and should follow the principles as in generally critically ill patients, but with some special considerations (**Table 5**).[3,64–66] Of note, an easy-to-

Table 5
Intensive care unit management of ALF

Cerebral edema and intracranial hypertension	Grade I/II encephalopathy • Consider transfer to liver transplant facility and listing for transplantation • CT brain: rule out other causes of altered mental status • Avoid stimulation; avoid sedation if possible • Lactulose, possibly helpful Grade III or IV encephalopathy • Continue management strategies listed above • Intubate trachea (may require sedation) • Elevate head of bed (~30°) • Consider placement of ICP monitoring device in selected cases • Immediate treatment of seizures required; prophylaxis of unclear value • Mannitol (0.25–1 g/kg IV bolus): use for severe elevation of ICP or first clinical signs of herniation • Hypertonic saline to increase serum sodium to 140–150 mmol/L • Hyperventilation: effects short lived; may use for impending herniation
Infections	• Surveillance for and prompt antimicrobial treatment of infection required (low threshold for empiric antibiotics if hemodynamic deterioration and/or increasing encephalopathy with inflammatory phenotype) • Antibiotic prophylaxis possibly helpful but not proven • Antifungal coverage for patients not responding to broad spectrum antibiotics and with infection/sepsis physiology
Bleeding and coagulopathy	• Vitamin K (10 mg IV or SC): give at least 1 dose • FFP: give only for invasive procedures or active bleeding • Cryoprecipitate: for fibrinogen <100 mg/dL and bleeding • Platelets: give only for invasive procedures or active bleeding • Hemoglobin target for transfusion is 7 g/dL • Recombinant activated factor VII (40 μg/kg bolus): possibly for invasive procedures (expensive and has a risk of thrombosis) • Prophylaxis for stress ulceration: give PPI or H2RA (consider stopping prophylaxis when feeding has been established)
Hemodynamics and renal failure	• Volume replacement • Vasopressor support (norepinephrine is the vasopressor of choice) as needed to maintain adequate MAP (target MAP ≥60–75 mm Hg) • Vasopressin or terlipressin recommended in hypotension refractory to volume resuscitation and norepinephrine (but should be used cautiously in patients with ICH) • Hydrocortisone therapy does not reduce mortality, but does decrease vasopressor requirements in patients with vasopressor resistant shock • Avoid nephrotoxic agents • Continuous modes of hemodialysis if needed
Pulmonary	• Sedation for endotracheal intubation and suctioning to prevent increased ICP • Ventilator management: tidal volumes 6 mL/kg, low PEEP
Metabolic Concerns	• Follow closely: glucose, potassium, magnesium, phosphate, lactate, blood gas • Glucose infusions (10%–20%): glycemic target ~140 mg/dL • Consider nutrition: enteral feedings if possible or total parenteral nutrition

(continued on next page)

Table 5 (continued)	
Extracorporeal liver support systems	• Should only be used in selected patients or within the context of a clinical trial • MARS and high-volume plasma exchange have been most studied in ALF

Abbreviations: ALF, acute liver failure; CT, computed tomography; FFP, fresh-frozen plasma; H2RA, histamine-2 receptor antagonists; ICH, intracranial hypertension; ICP, intracranial pressure; IV, intravenous; MAP, mean arterial blood pressure; MARS, molecular adsorbent recirculating system; PEEP, positive end-expiratory pressure; PPI, proton-pump inhibitors; SC, subcutaneously.

Data from Lee WM, Stravitz, Larson AM. AASLD position paper: the management of acute liver failure: update 2011. The American Association for the Study of Liver Diseases. Available at: https://www.aasld.org/sites/default/files/guideline_documents/alfenhanced.pdf and European Association for the Study of the Liver. J Hepatol 2017;66(5):1047–81.

use checklist for the management of ALF in the intensive care unit developed by the US-ALFSG is helpful and has been accepted by several centers in North America.[67]

Specific Treatment According to the Etiology

N-acetylcysteine (NAC), a glutathione precursor, is an established antidote for APAP poisoning and should be administered in all patients with APAP hepatotoxicity and APAP-induced ALF, and in those at significant risk for developing hepatotoxicity (based on the amount of APAP ingestion and/or serum APAP levels). Intravenous NAC has shown to improve LT-free survival by 20% to 30% among patients with APAP-induced ALF.[68,69] Apart from detoxifying *N*-acetyl-para-benzoquinoneimine, an intermediate metabolite of APAP, the potential mechanisms of NAC in this state include improving hepatic perfusion and oxygen delivery, scavenging reactive oxygen and nitrogen species, and refining mitochondrial energy production.[25] Intravenous administration (loading dose is 150 mg/kg in 5% dextrose over 15 minutes; maintenance dose is 50 mg/kg given over 4 hours followed by 100 mg/kg administered over 16 hours or 6 mg/kg/h) is recommended for patients with ALF. About 10% to 20% of patients may develop some side effects, such as nausea, vomiting, and anaphylactoid reactions.[3,25] Controversy exists over when to stop the use of NAC; whether a standard 72-hour period is optimal or continuation until liver chemistry values have improved is preferred.[3] The European Association for the Study of the Liver experts suggest that the use of NAC be limited to a maximum duration of 5 days, given its antiinflammatory effects, which are unlikely to be impacted and, further, may increase risk of infections in the later phase of ALF.[4]

The role of NAC for non–APAP-associated ALF has also been evaluated. In an randomized, controlled trial of intravenous NAC for non–APAP-associated ALF (n = 173), NAC did not improve LT-free survival at 3 weeks. However, a subanalysis revealed improved LT-free survival in 114 patients with early stage encephalopathy (grades I or II; 52% compared with 30% for placebo; *P* = .01).[70] In contrast, a multicenter, observational study of 155 patients with non–APAP-associated ALF from Egypt (85 were given NAC; 70 were not) reported that NAC significantly reduced mortality (LT-free survival: 96.4% vs 23.3%; *P*<.01), need for LT, and encephalopathy.[71] In a randomized, controlled trial in non–APAP-associated ALF in pediatric patients (n = 184), NAC did not improve 1-year survival and, in addition, noted a lower LT-free survival among those less than 2 years of age.[72]

Corticosteroids have been proposed as a potential therapeutic intervention for patients with ALF owing to autoimmune hepatitis, hypersensitivity drug reaction, and Epstein-Barr virus based on a presumed immune-mediated pathogenesis.[21,29,73,74]

In a retrospective analysis of 361 patients with ALF (66 with autoimmune etiology, 164 with indeterminate etiology, and 131 with drug-induced ALF) in the US-ASLFG from 1998 to 2007, corticosteroid use was not associated with improved overall survival (61% vs 66%; $P = .41$), nor with improved survival in any diagnosis category. Further, the use of corticosteroid was associated with diminished survival in those with very high MELD score (>40; survival of 30% vs 57%; $P = .03$).[75] Despite the lack of demonstrable benefit of anti-HBV therapy in the US-ALFSG HBV-induced ALF cohort, potent nucleos(t)ide analogues should be strongly considered in all patients with HBV-induced ALF (also impending ALF), particularly in LT candidates. Viral suppression may potentially help recovery and, if LT is necessary, it likely will prevent HBV recurrence after grafting.[76,77]

Hepatic Encephalopathy and Cerebral Edema

Cerebral edema (CE) and intracranial hypertension (ICH) have long been recognized as cardinal features and major causes of death in ALF (brainstem herniation). These manifestations may also contribute to ischemic and hypoxic brain injury, which may result in long-term neurologic deficits in survivors.[3] The incidence of CE and ICH has been decreasing over the time and may reflect improvements in the preventive care and use of early LT. However, once CE has developed in ALF, it is still associated with very poor survival and thus complex critical care management is required.[6,9]

The pathogenesis of CE and ICH in ALF is multifactorial and includes hyperammonia (causing accumulation of glutamine within astrocytes, which leads to an osmotic stress and cytotoxic edema), loss of cerebrovascular autoregulation, neuroinflammation, systemic inflammatory response syndrome, disruption of the blood–brain barrier (causing vasogenic edema), endothelial dysfunction, and other contributing causes (eg, metabolic disturbances, medications, and hypoxia).[3,6,78,79] The strong risk factors for CE and ICH in ALF are severity of HE (ICH in 25%–35% with HE grade III and >65%–75% with HE grade IV) and duration of illness (highest with hyperacute liver failure where >70% developed ICH).[3,5,80] Other risk factors include female gender, young age, acute renal failure, and requirement for vasopressors and renal replacement therapy.[3,9,81] Blood ammonia levels, preferably arterial, may also be helpful; levels greater than 150 to 200 μmol/L have been shown to correlate with CE and ICH, whereas levels less than 75 μmol/L may preclude the development of severe HE or ICH.[81,82] The blood sample should be drawn without using a tourniquet and transported within 20 minutes of the blood draw on ice.[83]

CE and ICH should be suspected clinically in patients with ALF with new-onset systemic hypertension, bradycardia, progression of hyperventilation and encephalopathy, alterations in pupillary and oculovestibular reflexes, myoclonus, or decerebration.[3,79,80] However, most of these clinical signs are not specific or sensitive and may evolve in patients even in those with grade IV HE and without ICH.[80] Non–contrast-enhanced computed tomography scanning is often performed mainly to exclude intracranial pathology, particularly bleeding. Features of CE with or without signs of herniation may be observed on computed tomography scans (**Fig. 1**); however, the absence of these findings does not exclude CE and ICH, especially at the early stages.[3,79,80]

The use of intracranial pressure (ICP) monitoring devices in patients with ALF remains controversial, and practices vary widely among centers. A survey performed among 24 LT centers in the US-ALFSG revealed that ICP monitoring device was used in 92 of 322 patients (28%) with ALF and severe HE from 1998 to 2004. Intracranial hemorrhage occurred in 10.3% (one-half of these complications were incidental radiologic findings) and the 30-day survival after LT was similar in both the monitored

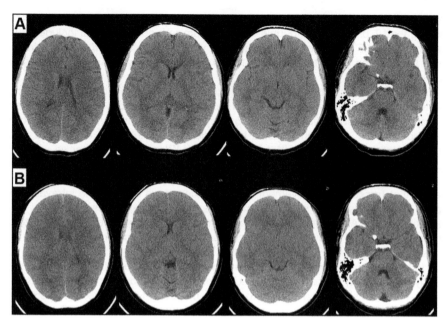

Fig. 1. (*A*) Computed tomography (CT) scan of the brain of a patient with acute liver failure and grade III encephalopathy showed mild cerebral edema with loss of sulci and gyri, blurring of grey-white junctions and mild narrowing of ventricles. (*B*) CT of the brain of the same patient (5 days later) showed progression of cerebral edema and impending brain herniation.

and the nonmonitored cohorts (85% vs 85%).[84] In Europe, there has been heterogeneity in the use of ICP monitoring in ALF; greater than 60% at King's College Hospital, 20% to 30% in Birmingham (UK) and Copenhagen, approximately 16% in Spain, and usually not used in France.[85] The main rationale for monitoring ICP is to allow assessment of cerebral perfusion pressure (CPP; calculated as the mean arterial pressure [MAP] minus the ICP), to avoid cerebral hypoperfusion during ICH by targeting CPP at greater than 60 mm Hg and ICP to less than 20 mm Hg either by administering osmotically active agents and/or vasopressors.[3] In addition, refractory ICH and/or decreased CPP may be considered relative contraindications for LT because of concern about poor neurologic recovery.[3,85] The European Association for the Study of the Liver guideline recommends that invasive ICP monitoring be considered in highly selected subgroup of patients with grade III or IV coma, who are mechanically ventilated and deemed at high risk of ICH based on the presence of more than 1 of the following criteria: (1) young patients with hyperacute or acute ALF, (2) an ammonia level greater than 150 to 200 μmol/L that does not decrease with initial treatment interventions, (3) renal impairment, and (4) vasopressor support (>1.0 μg/kg/min).[4] Noninvasive assessments of ICP and CPP, such as transcranial Doppler ultrasonography,[83,86] ocular ultrasonography,[83,87] and near-infrared spectrophotometry,[88] have also been evaluated in patients with ALF, but their use is center specific and guidelines on their use consistently across various centers have not been harmonized.

Patients with mild HE may benefit with lactulose as suggested in a retrospective study from the US-ALFSG (increased median survival time from 7 to 15 days while awaiting LT without changes in mortality or need for LT).[89] Caution is to be exercised in the overuse of lactulose because the pathogenic mechanisms of HE differ in ALF from those with chronic liver disease; further overuse may lead to bowel dilation challenging the LT procedure. A double-blind, randomized, controlled trial included 201 patients with ALF (mainly owing to hepatitis E virus) demonstrated that L-ornithine L-aspartate infusion did not lower ammonia, or improve the level of consciousness or survival.[90]

As patients progress to grade III or IV encephalopathy, intubation and mechanical ventilation are mandatory.[3] Small doses of propofol may be used for sedation because it may reduce cerebral blood flow. As prophylactic measures to reduce the risk of development of ICH, patients should be positioned with the head elevated at 30°, and stimulation and pain should be minimized.[3] If ICH develops, either as seen on ICP monitoring or by obvious neurologic signs, osmotic agents such as mannitol are often effective in decreasing ICH by creating a gradient across the blood–brain barrier that forces water movement from the edematous brain to the intravascular space. Mannitol has been shown in small series to correct episodes of elevated ICP in patients with ALF, and also to improve survival (supported by a randomized, controlled trial).[3,80,91] However, its effect is short lived, and may not be effective for patients with severe ICH (ICP >60 mm Hg).[3,64,80,91] The dose may be repeated as needed if the serum osmolality is less than 320 mOsm/L. Potential adverse events are hyperosmolarity, hypernatremia, and volume overload for which the patients be closely monitored.[3] Hyperventilation to a $Paco_2$ of 25 to 30 mm Hg restores cerebrovascular autoregulation, resulting in vasoconstriction and reduction of ICP. If severe ICH is not controlled with mannitol, hyperventilation may be instituted acutely to delay impending herniation.[3,64,80] However, the effect of hyperventilation on cerebral blood flow is transient and there has been some concern that vasoconstriction may cause cerebral hypoxia. A randomized, controlled trial of prophylactic continuous hyperventilation in patients with ALF revealed no reduction in the incidence of CE and ICH and no survival benefit, although onset of cerebral herniation seemed to be delayed in the hyperventilated group.[92]

Based on studies in patients with traumatic brain injury, hypertonic saline boluses have been found to have a similar or even superior efficacy to mannitol.[93,94] In a randomized, controlled trial of patients with ALF and grade III or IV encephalopathy (n = 30), prophylactic induction of hypernatremia (aim for serum sodium of 145–155 mEq/L for 72 hours) with 30% hypertonic saline reduced the incidence and severity of ICH compared with normonatremic standard of care.[95] Although a survival benefit with induced hypernatremia was not demonstrated, the American Association for the Study of Liver Diseases Practice Guideline recommends the use of hypertonic saline as a prophylactic measure in patients at greatest risk of developing CE and ICH.[3] However, serum sodium greater than 150 mmol/L may be associated with cell damage and should be avoided. Therefore, hypertonic saline infusions should be targeted to maintain serum sodium at 140 to 145 mmol/L.[4] There has been no study that evaluated hypertonic saline as a treatment for established ICH in ALF. Therapeutic hypothermia (cooling to core temperature of 33°C–34°C) may prevent or control ICH in patients with ALF, but its potential harmful effects include increased risk of infection, coagulation disturbance, arrhythmias, and reduced liver regeneration.[3,96] Although 2 uncontrolled studies from the UK suggested some benefits of hypothermia in ALF,[97,98] a subsequent randomized, controlled trial of moderate hypothermia in patients with ALF and grade III or IV encephalopathy (n = 46) found no benefit on improving survival or preventing ICH.[99] Similarly, a retrospective analysis from the US-ALFSG (97/1232 patients received therapeutic hypothermia) found no survival benefit from moderate hypothermia, although a survival benefit was observed in young patients (<25 years of age) with APAP-associated ALF.[100]

In situations where the patient has cerebral hyperemia and signs of ICH persist despite mannitol and hypertonic saline, a bolus of intravenous indomethacin may be considered.[4,101]

Seizures increase ICP and should be controlled promptly with short-acting benzodiazepines plus phenytoin or levetiracetam. Although seizure activity in patients with ALF can be subclinical, the prophylactic use of phenytoin is not recommended currently, because available randomized, controlled trials have shown conflicting results.[102,103]

Infections

Patients with ALF have an increased susceptibility for infections as a result of excessive systemic inflammation, mainly from cytokine storm, multiple organ dysfunction, and functional immunoparesis, particularly impaired function of leukocytes, macrophages, and complement systems.[104,105] Risks of infection are further amplified by the presence of indwelling lines, catheters, and tubes.[104,105] Microbial infections have been documented in up to 80% of ALF cases; approximately 50% pneumonia, 15% to 26% bacteremia, and approximately 30% fungal infections (mainly candidiasis).[106–108]

The classic signs of infection such as fever and leukocytosis, however, can be absent in up to 30% of patients with ALF.[105,108] In addition, although serum procalcitonin seems to be a helpful assay for detecting bacterial infections in general, there has been poor discrimination between patients with ALF with or without bacterial infection, presumably because of the massive liver injury.[109] Sepsis leads to negative outcomes among patients with ALF. Bacteremia and systemic inflammatory response syndrome are associated with an increased severity of HE, coagulopathy, and renal failure.[105] Sepsis can affect the outcome of LT adversely, and increases mortality in patients with ALF, with the reported attributable mortality ranging from 10% to 52%.[105–107]

Although prophylactic antimicrobial therapy reduces the incidence of infection in certain groups of patients with ALF, prophylactic antibiotics and antifungals have not been shown to improve overall outcomes in ALF and, therefore, cannot be advocated in all patients, particularly those with mild HE.[3,105,106] Strict implementation of infection prevention control measures and periodic surveillance for infections (eg, chest radiography and periodic cultures of sputum, urine, and blood for fungal and bacterial organisms) should be undertaken. Antibiotics should be initiated promptly based on surveillance culture results, or at the earliest clinical signs of active infection or clinical deterioration.[3,4,105]

Acute Kidney Injury

AKI develops in 56% to 70% of patients with ALF and has been associated with decreased short-term and long-term overall survival.[110,111] AKI is often multifactorial, and is more common with certain etiologies, including ischemic hepatitis, Wilson disease, acute fatty liver of pregnancy, HELLP (hemolysis, elevated liver enzymes, low platelets) syndrome, heat stroke, hepatitis A virus, *Amanita* poisoning, or hepatotoxicity owing to APAP, phenytoin, trimethoprim–sulfamethoxazole, or macrolides.[64,111] Most patients with ALF with AKI fully recover renal function either after LT or spontaneously.[4] Renal replacement therapy is required in approximately 30% of cases and the classic indications including severe acidosis, hyperkalemia, and/or fluid overload. Additional indications include the removal of toxic substances, and difficult to treat hyponatremia or hyperthermia.[64,110] Continuous modes of renal replacement therapy are preferred because they have been shown in a randomized, controlled trial to result in improved stability in cardiovascular and intracranial parameters compared with intermittent modes.[3,4,112]

Extracorporeal Liver Support Systems

The rationale for using an extracorporeal liver support system (ELSS) in ALF is to help maintain homeostasis while the liver regenerates or until an organ is available for LT. Several strategies have been developed to remove toxins and maintain biosynthesis, which can broadly be divided into artificial and bioartificial liver support systems.[64,113] Artificial support systems are cell-free systems that can be subdivided further into conventional extracorporeal procedures (eg, hemodialysis, hemofiltration, plasmapheresis, and hemodiabsorption) and albumin dialysis (eg, molecular adsorbent recirculating system [MARS], single pass albumin dialysis, or fractionated plasma separation and adsorption [Prometheus; Fresenius Medical Care, Bad Homburg vor der Höhe, Germany]). Bioartificial systems incorporate hepatocytes, with or without the artificial systems described, include the extracorporeal liver assist device, which uses aggregates from C3a hepatoma cell lines, and HepatAssist (AirBios Systems, Inc, Waltham, MA), which uses porcine hepatocytes together with a charcoal column.[41,113]

Among several techniques reported, only 2 artificial ELSS have been studied in ALF with well-designed randomized, controlled trials, namely MARS and high-volume plasma exchange (HVP). In a randomized, controlled trial in France (n = 102), MARS has not been shown to improve 6-month survival in ALF (75.5% with conventional treatment vs 82.9% with MARS in the per-protocol population; $P = .50$). However, a confounder may have been the short median listing to LT time, which was only 16 hours (75% of enrolled patients underwent LT within 24 hours).[114] A recent metaanalysis of 11 trials (n = 781 patients) evaluating ELSS in ALF and acute-on-chronic liver failure showed a statistically significant improvement in overall survival (relative risk [RR], 0.86; 95% CI, 0.74–1.00).[41] When focusing on ALF (7 trials involving 415 patients), there was no improvement in survival in the artificial support system group (RR, 0.86; 95% CI, 0.70–1.06).[20,30–34] Five randomized, controlled trials reported that adverse events were similar between the ELSS and usual care, but 1 randomized, controlled trial found that 2 of 12 patients randomized to an extracorporeal liver assist device withdrew owing to fever and bleeding.[41,115] In a post hoc analysis looking at trials within the past 20 years in ALF (presumably techniques have improved and patient populations different), there was a marginally statistically significant benefit of artificial support systems in 4 trials (RR, 0.75; 95% CI, 0.57–0.99).[114–117] Four randomized, controlled trials (n = 228) assessing traditional extracorporeal methods showed no decrease in mortality (RR, 0.94; 95% CI, 0.74–1.20). Four randomized, controlled trials (n = 340) assessing MARS compared with usual care showed no statistically significant decrease in mortality with MARS, although there was a trend to benefit (RR, 0.79; 95% CI, 0.60–1.06).[41]

It should be noted that there was a subsequent randomized, controlled trial (n = 182) evaluating HVP versus standard medical therapy in ALF, which was not included in the aforementioned metaanalysis.[118] In this randomized, controlled trial, treatment with HVP (15% of ideal body weight representing 8–12 L/d for 3 days) improved outcome in patients with ALF by increasing LT-free survival (overall hospital survival, 58.7% vs 47.8%; hazard ratio, 0.56; 95% CI, 0.36–0.86; $P = .0083$).[118] In those who underwent LT (n = 56), HVP did not improve survival compared with standard medical therapy alone ($P = .75$). A parallel proof-of-principle study demonstrated that HVP attenuates innate immune activation and ameliorates multiorgan dysfunction.[118] Therefore, HVP may be of greater benefit in patients who are treated early and thus ultimately may be able to avoid undergoing LT.[4] In summary, the overall benefits of ELSS in ALF remain uncertain. ELSS may reduce overall and LT-free survival in select patients, but also may harm in some and therefore ELSS should not be routinely used in ALF until more data became available.

Liver Transplantation

Urgent LT is the only definitive treatment for patients with ALF when prognostic indicators suggest a high likelihood of death. Decisions to list and transplant must be made early in all patients with ALF, particularly in those with APAP-associated failure in whom ALF outcomes evolve rapidly, and where they either survive without LT or die.[119] Overall 1-year survival after LT has been reported to be lower for patients with ALF in comparison to patients with cirrhosis (most deaths after LT for ALF occur within the first 3 months from infections and neurologic complications); however, after the first year this trend has been to be reversed and patients with ALF have a better long-term survival.[120–122] Nevertheless, the 21-day survival rate after LT for ALF has significantly improved over the past 16 years: from 88.3% to 96.3% ($P<.01$).[8] ALF is one of few conditions for which a patient can be listed as a United Network for Organ Sharing status 1A (urgent) in the United States and "super urgent" in the UK.[3] Based on the largest series from US-ALFSG, of 617 patients with ALF listed for LT (36% of overall ALF), 117 (19%) spontaneously survived, 108 (17.5%) died without LT, and 392 (63.5%) underwent LT.[119] Cadaveric donor LT has been the standard in ALF, but living-donor or auxiliary LT may also be considered if organ support is limited, although its use remains controversial and should be done only in large-volume centers.[3,64,123,124] The use of ABO-incompatible grafts showed less favorable outcomes (30%–60% 1-year graft survival).[125,126]

REFERENCES

1. O'Grady JG, Schalm SW, Williams R. Acute liver failure: redefining the syndromes. Lancet 1993;342(8866):273–5.
2. Tandon BN, Bernauau J, O'Grady J, et al. Recommendations of the International Association for the study of the liver subcommittee on nomenclature of acute and subacute liver failure. J Gastroenterol Hepatol 1999;14(5):403–4.
3. Lee WM, Stravitz RT, Larson AM. Introduction to the revised American Association for the Study of Liver Diseases position paper on acute liver failure 2011. Hepatology 2012;55(3):965–7.
4. European Association for the Study of the Liver. EASL Clinical Practical Guidelines on the management of acute (fulminant) liver failure. J Hepatol 2017;66(5): 1047–81.
5. Tujios SR, Lee WM. Acute liver failure. In: Dooley JS, Lok ASF, Burroughs AK, et al, editors. Sherlock's diseases of the liver and biliary system. 12th edition. Oxford (United Kingdom): Blackwell Publishing; 2011.
6. Bernal W, Lee WM, Wendon J, et al. Acute liver failure: a curable disease by 2024? J Hepatol 2015;62(1 Suppl):S112–20.
7. Chung RT, Stravitz RT, Fontana RJ, et al. Pathogenesis of liver injury in acute liver failure. Gastroenterology 2012;143(3):e1–7.
8. Reuben A, Tillman H, Fontana RJ, et al. Outcomes in adults with acute liver failure between 1998 and 2013: an observational cohort study. Ann Intern Med 2016;164(11):724–32.
9. Bernal W, Hyyrylainen A, Gera A, et al. Lessons from look-back in acute liver failure? A single centre experience of 3300 patients. J Hepatol 2013;59(1):74–80.
10. Ichai P, Samuel D. Etiology and prognosis of fulminant hepatitis in adults. Liver Transpl 2008;14(Suppl 2):S67–79.

11. Lee WM. Etiologies of acute liver failure. Semin Liver Dis 2008;28(2):142–52.

12. Hadem J, Tacke F, Bruns T, et al. Etiologies and outcomes of acute liver failure in Germany. Clin Gastroenterol Hepatol 2012;10(6):664–9.e2.

13. Mas A, Escorsell A, Fernandez J. Liver transplantation for acute liver failure: a Spanish perspective. Transplant Proc 2010;42(2):619–21.

14. Oketani M, Ido A, Tsubouchi H. Changing etiologies and outcomes of acute liver failure: a perspective from Japan. J Gastroenterol Hepatol 2011;26(Suppl 1): 65–71.

15. Bunchorntavakul C, Reddy KR. Drug hepatotoxicity: newer agents. Clin Liver Dis 2017;21(1):115–34.

16. Bunchorntavakul C, Reddy KR. Review article: herbal and dietary supplement hepatotoxicity. Aliment Pharmacol Ther 2013;37(1):3–17.

17. Fontana RJ, Engle RE, Scaglione S, et al. The role of hepatitis E virus infection in adult Americans with acute liver failure. Hepatology 2016;64(6):1870–80.

18. Shalimar, Kedia S, Gunjan D, et al. Acute liver failure due to hepatitis e virus infection is associated with better survival than other etiologies in Indian patients. Dig Dis Sci 2017;62(4):1058–66.

19. Rezende G, Roque-Afonso AM, Samuel D, et al. Viral and clinical factors associated with the fulminant course of hepatitis A infection. Hepatology 2003;38(3): 613–8.

20. Taylor RM, Davern T, Munoz S, et al. Fulminant hepatitis A virus infection in the United States: incidence, prognosis, and outcomes. Hepatology 2006;44(6): 1589–97.

21. Mellinger JL, Rossaro L, Naugler WE, et al. Epstein-Barr virus (EBV) related acute liver failure: a case series from the US Acute Liver Failure Study Group. Dig Dis Sci 2014;59(7):1630–7.

22. Karvellas CJ, Cardoso FS, Gottfried M, et al. HBV-associated acute liver failure after immunosuppression and risk of death. Clin Gastroenterol Hepatol 2017; 15(1):113–22.

23. Ichai P, Roque Afonso AM, Sebagh M, et al. Herpes simplex virus-associated acute liver failure: a difficult diagnosis with a poor prognosis. Liver Transpl 2005;11(12):1550–5.

24. Norvell JP, Blei AT, Jovanovic BD, et al. Herpes simplex virus hepatitis: an analysis of the published literature and institutional cases. Liver Transpl 2007;13(10): 1428–34.

25. Bunchorntavakul C, Reddy KR. Acetaminophen-related hepatotoxicity. Clin Liver Dis 2013;17(4):587–607, viii.

26. Hillman L, Gottfried M, Whitsett M, et al. Clinical features and outcomes of complementary and alternative medicine induced acute liver failure and injury. Am J Gastroenterol 2016;111(7):958–65.

27. Reuben A, Koch DG, Lee WM. Drug-induced acute liver failure: results of a U.S. multicenter, prospective study. Hepatology 2010;52(6):2065–76.

28. Stravitz RT, Lefkowitch JH, Fontana RJ, et al. Autoimmune acute liver failure: proposed clinical and histological criteria. Hepatology 2011;53(2):517–26.

29. Verma S, Maheshwari A, Thuluvath P. Liver failure as initial presentation of autoimmune hepatitis: clinical characteristics, predictors of response to steroid therapy, and outcomes. Hepatology 2009;49(4):1396–7.

30. Dhawan A, Taylor RM, Cheeseman P, et al. Wilson's disease in children: 37-year experience and revised King's score for liver transplantation. Liver Transpl 2005; 11(4):441–8.

31. Escudie L, Francoz C, Vinel JP, et al. Amanita phalloides poisoning: reassessment of prognostic factors and indications for emergency liver transplantation. J Hepatol 2007;46(3):466–73.

32. Ganzert M, Felgenhauer N, Zilker T. Indication of liver transplantation following amatoxin intoxication. J Hepatol 2005;42(2):202–9.

33. Karvellas CJ, Tillman H, Leung AA, et al. Acute liver injury and acute liver failure from mushroom poisoning in North America. Liver Int 2016;36(7):1043–50.

34. Bonacini M, Shetler K, Yu I, et al. Features of patients with severe hepatitis due to mushroom poisoning and factors associated with outcome. Clin Gastroenterol Hepatol 2017;15(5):776–9.

35. Taylor RM, Tujios S, Jinjuvadia K, et al. Short and long-term outcomes in patients with acute liver failure due to ischemic hepatitis. Dig Dis Sci 2012;57(3):777–85.

36. Parekh J, Matei VM, Canas-Coto A, et al. Budd-Chiari syndrome causing acute liver failure: a multicenter case series. Liver Transpl 2017;23(2):135–42.

37. James LP, Letzig L, Simpson PM, et al. Pharmacokinetics of acetaminophen-protein adducts in adults with acetaminophen overdose and acute liver failure. Drug Metab Dispos 2009;37(8):1779–84.

38. Roberts DW, Lee WM, Hinson JA, et al. An immunoassay to rapidly measure acetaminophen protein adducts accurately identifies patients with acute liver injury or failure. Clin Gastroenterol Hepatol 2017;15(4):555–62.e3.

39. Khandelwal N, James LP, Sanders C, et al. Unrecognized acetaminophen toxicity as a cause of indeterminate acute liver failure. Hepatology 2011;53(2): 567–76.

40. Flamm SL, Yang YX, Singh S, et al. American Gastroenterological Association Institute Guidelines for the diagnosis and management of acute liver failure. Gastroenterology 2017;152(3):644–7.

41. Herrine SK, Moayyedi P, Brown RS Jr, et al. American Gastroenterological Association Institute technical review on initial testing and management of acute liver disease. Gastroenterology 2017;152(3):648–64.e5.

42. Ostapowicz G, Fontana RJ, Schiodt FV, et al. Results of a prospective study of acute liver failure at 17 tertiary care centers in the United States. Ann Intern Med 2002;137(12):947–54.

43. O'Grady JG, Alexander GJ, Hayllar KM, et al. Early indicators of prognosis in fulminant hepatic failure. Gastroenterology 1989;97(2):439–45.

44. Fontana RJ, Ellerbe C, Durkalski VE, et al. Two-year outcomes in initial survivors with acute liver failure: results from a prospective, multicentre study. Liver Int 2015;35(2):370–80.

45. Cholongitas E, Senzolo M, Patch D, et al. Review article: scoring systems for assessing prognosis in critically ill adult cirrhotics. Aliment Pharmacol Ther 2006; 24(3):453–64.

46. McPhail MJ, Wendon JA, Bernal W. Meta-analysis of performance of Kings's College Hospital criteria in prediction of outcome in non-paracetamol-induced acute liver failure. J Hepatol 2010;53(3):492–9.

47. Bernal W, Donaldson N, Wyncoll D, et al. Blood lactate as an early predictor of outcome in paracetamol-induced acute liver failure: a cohort study. Lancet 2002;359(9306):558–63.

48. Zaman MB, Hoti E, Qasim A, et al. MELD score as a prognostic model for listing acute liver failure patients for liver transplantation. Transplant Proc 2006;38(7): 2097–8.

49. Bernuau J, Rueff B, Benhamou JP. Fulminant and subfulminant liver failure: definitions and causes. Semin Liver Dis 1986;6(2):97–106.

50. Izumi S, Langley PG, Wendon J, et al. Coagulation factor V levels as a prognostic indicator in fulminant hepatic failure. Hepatology 1996;23(6):1507–11.

51. Pereira LM, Langley PG, Hayllar KM, et al. Coagulation factor V and VIII/V ratio as predictors of outcome in paracetamol induced fulminant hepatic failure: relation to other prognostic indicators. Gut 1992;33(1):98–102.

52. Mitchell I, Bihari D, Chang R, et al. Earlier identification of patients at risk from acetaminophen-induced acute liver failure. Crit Care Med 1998;26(2):279–84.

53. Koch DG, Tillman H, Durkalski V, et al. Development of a model to predict transplant-free survival of patients with acute liver failure. Clin Gastroenterol Hepatol 2016;14(8):1199–206.e2.

54. Schmidt LE, Dalhoff K. Alpha-fetoprotein is a predictor of outcome in acetaminophen-induced liver injury. Hepatology 2005;41(1):26–31.

55. Schiodt FV, Bondesen S, Petersen I, et al. Admission levels of serum Gc-globulin: predictive value in fulminant hepatic failure. Hepatology 1996;23(4):713–8.

56. Schmidt LE, Dalhoff K. Serum phosphate is an early predictor of outcome in severe acetaminophen-induced hepatotoxicity. Hepatology 2002;36(3):659–65.

57. Rosen HR, Biggins SW, Niki T, et al. Association between plasma level of Galectin-9 and survival of patients with drug-induced acute liver failure. Clin Gastroenterol Hepatol 2016;14(4):606–12.e3.

58. Stravitz RT, Bowling R, Bradford RL, et al. Role of procoagulant microparticles in mediating complications and outcome of acute liver injury/acute liver failure. Hepatology 2013;58(1):304–13.

59. Moller HJ, Gronbaek H, Schiodt FV, et al. Soluble CD163 from activated macrophages predicts mortality in acute liver failure. J Hepatol 2007;47(5):671–6.

60. Karvellas CJ, Speiser JL, Tremblay M, et al. Elevated FABP1 serum levels are associated with poorer survival in acetaminophen-induced acute liver failure. Hepatology 2017;65(3):938–49.

61. Robles-Diaz M, Lucena MI, Kaplowitz N, et al. Use of Hy's law and a new composite algorithm to predict acute liver failure in patients with drug-induced liver injury. Gastroenterology 2014;147(1):109–18.e5.

62. Lo Re V 3rd, Haynes K, Forde KA, et al. Risk of acute liver failure in patients with drug-induced liver injury: evaluation of Hy's law and a new prognostic model. Clin Gastroenterol Hepatol 2015;13(13):2360–8.

63. Koch DG, Speiser JL, Durkalski V, et al. The natural history of severe acute liver injury. Am J Gastroenterol 2017. [Epub ahead of print].

64. Cardoso FS, Marcelino P, Bagulho L, et al. Acute liver failure: an up-to-date approach. J Crit Care 2017;39:25–30.

65. Siddiqui MS, Stravitz RT. Intensive care unit management of patients with liver failure. Clin Liver Dis 2014;18(4):957–78.

66. Stravitz RT, Kramer AH, Davern T, et al. Intensive care of patients with acute liver failure: recommendations of the U.S. Acute Liver Failure Study Group. Crit Care Med 2007;35(11):2498–508.

67. Fix OK, Liou I, Karvellas CJ, et al. Development and pilot of a checklist for management of acute liver failure in the intensive care unit. PLoS One 2016;11(5):e0155500.

68. Harrison PM, Keays R, Bray GP, et al. Improved outcome of paracetamol-induced fulminant hepatic failure by late administration of acetylcysteine. Lancet 1990;335(8705):1572–3.

69. Keays R, Harrison PM, Wendon JA, et al. Intravenous acetylcysteine in paracet-amol induced fulminant hepatic failure: a prospective controlled trial. BMJ 1991; 303(6809):1026–9.

70. Lee WM, Hynan LS, Rossaro L, et al. Intravenous N-acetylcysteine improves transplant-free survival in early stage non-acetaminophen acute liver failure. Gastroenterology 2009;137(3):856–64, 864.e1.

71. Darweesh SK, Ibrahim MF, El-Tahawy MA. Effect of N-Acetylcysteine on mortal-ity and liver transplantation rate in non-acetaminophen-induced acute liver fail-ure: a multicenter study. Clin Drug Investig 2017;37(5):473–82.

72. Squires RH, Dhawan A, Alonso E, et al. Intravenous N-acetylcysteine in pediat-ric patients with nonacetaminophen acute liver failure: a placebo-controlled clin-ical trial. Hepatology 2013;57(4):1542–9.

73. Randomised trial of steroid therapy in acute liver failure. Report from the Euro-pean Association for the Study of the Liver (EASL). Gut 1979;20(7):620–3.

74. Rakela J, Mosley JW, Edwards VM, et al. A double-blinded, randomized trial of hydrocortisone in acute hepatic failure. The Acute Hepatic Failure Study Group. Dig Dis Sci 1991;36(9):1223–8.

75. Karkhanis J, Verna EC, Chang MS, et al. Steroid use in acute liver failure. Hep-atology 2014;59(2):612–21.

76. Dao DY, Seremba E, Ajmera V, et al. Use of nucleoside (tide) analogues in pa-tients with hepatitis B-related acute liver failure. Dig Dis Sci 2012;57(5):1349–57.

77. Sarin SK, Kumar M, Lau GK, et al. Asian-Pacific clinical practice guidelines on the management of hepatitis B: a 2015 update. Hepatol Int 2016;10(1):1–98.

78. Bosoi CR, Rose CF. Brain edema in acute liver failure and chronic liver disease: similarities and differences. Neurochem Int 2013;62(4):446–57.

79. Ryan JM, Tranah T, Mitry RR, et al. Acute liver failure and the brain: a look through the crystal ball. Metab Brain Dis 2013;28(1):7–10.

80. Mohsenin V. Assessment and management of cerebral edema and intracranial hypertension in acute liver failure. J Crit Care 2013;28(5):783–91.

81. Bernal W, Hall C, Karvellas CJ, et al. Arterial ammonia and clinical risk factors for encephalopathy and intracranial hypertension in acute liver failure. Hepatology 2007;46(6):1844–52.

82. Bhatia V, Singh R, Acharya SK. Predictive value of arterial ammonia for compli-cations and outcome in acute liver failure. Gut 2006;55(1):98–104.

83. Kodali S, McGuire BM. Diagnosis and management of hepatic encephalopathy in fulminant hepatic failure. Clin Liver Dis 2015;19(3):565–76.

84. Vaquero J, Fontana RJ, Larson AM, et al. Complications and use of intracranial pressure monitoring in patients with acute liver failure and severe encephalop-athy. Liver Transpl 2005;11(12):1581–9.

85. Bernuau J, Durand F. Intracranial pressure monitoring in patients with acute liver failure: a questionable invasive surveillance. Hepatology 2006;44(2):502–4.

86. Aggarwal S, Brooks DM, Kang Y, et al. Noninvasive monitoring of cerebral perfu-sion pressure in patients with acute liver failure using transcranial doppler ultra-sonography. Liver Transpl 2008;14(7):1048–57.

87. Kim YK, Seo H, Yu J, et al. Noninvasive estimation of raised intracranial pressure using ocular ultrasonography in liver transplant recipients with acute liver failure -A report of two cases. Korean J Anesthesiol 2013;64(5):451–5.

88. Nielsen HB, Tofteng F, Wang LP, et al. Cerebral oxygenation determined by near-infrared spectrophotometry in patients with fulminant hepatic failure. J Hepatol 2003;38(2):188–92.

89. Alba L, Hay JE, Angulo P, et al. Lactulose therapy in acute liver failure. J Hepatol 2002;36(suppl 1):33A.

90. Acharya SK, Bhatia V, Sreenivas V, et al. Efficacy of L-ornithine L-aspartate in acute liver failure: a double-blind, randomized, placebo-controlled study. Gastroenterology 2009;136(7):2159–68.

91. Canalese J, Gimson AE, Davis C, et al. Controlled trial of dexamethasone and mannitol for the cerebral oedema of fulminant hepatic failure. Gut 1982;23(7): 625–9.

92. Ede RJ, Gimson AE, Bihari D, et al. Controlled hyperventilation in the prevention of cerebral oedema in fulminant hepatic failure. J Hepatol 1986;2(1):43–51.

93. Battison C, Andrews PJ, Graham C, et al. Randomized, controlled trial on the effect of a 20% mannitol solution and a 7.5% saline/6% dextran solution on increased intracranial pressure after brain injury. Crit Care Med 2005;33(1): 196–202 [discussion: 257–8].

94. Ware ML, Nemani VM, Meeker M, et al. Effects of 23.4% sodium chloride solution in reducing intracranial pressure in patients with traumatic brain injury: a preliminary study. Neurosurgery 2005;57(4):727–36 [discussion: 727–36].

95. Murphy N, Auzinger G, Bernel W, et al. The effect of hypertonic sodium chloride on intracranial pressure in patients with acute liver failure. Hepatology 2004; 39(2):464–70.

96. Rose C, Michalak A, Pannunzio M, et al. Mild hypothermia delays the onset of coma and prevents brain edema and extracellular brain glutamate accumulation in rats with acute liver failure. Hepatology 2000;31(4):872–7.

97. Jalan R, Olde Damink SW, Deutz NE, et al. Moderate hypothermia prevents cerebral hyperemia and increase in intracranial pressure in patients undergoing liver transplantation for acute liver failure. Transplantation 2003;75(12):2034–9.

98. Jalan R, Olde Damink SW, Deutz NE, et al. Moderate hypothermia in patients with acute liver failure and uncontrolled intracranial hypertension. Gastroenterology 2004;127(5):1338–46.

99. Bernal W, Murphy N, Brown S, et al. A multicentre randomized controlled trial of moderate hypothermia to prevent intracranial hypertension in acute liver failure. J Hepatol 2016;65(2):273–9.

100. Karvellas CJ, Todd Stravitz R, Battenhouse H, et al. Therapeutic hypothermia in acute liver failure: a multicenter retrospective cohort analysis. Liver Transpl 2015;21(1):4–12.

101. Tofteng F, Larsen FS. The effect of indomethacin on intracranial pressure, cerebral perfusion and extracellular lactate and glutamate concentrations in patients with fulminant hepatic failure. J Cereb Blood Flow Metab 2004;24(7):798–804.

102. Bhatia V, Batra Y, Acharya SK. Prophylactic phenytoin does not improve cerebral edema or survival in acute liver failure–a controlled clinical trial. J Hepatol 2004;41(1):89–96.

103. Ellis AJ, Wendon JA, Williams R. Subclinical seizure activity and prophylactic phenytoin infusion in acute liver failure: a controlled clinical trial. Hepatology 2000;32(3):536–41.

104. Antoniades CG, Berry PA, Wendon JA, et al. The importance of immune dysfunction in determining outcome in acute liver failure. J Hepatol 2008; 49(5):845–61.

105. Dharel N, Bajaj JS. Antibiotic prophylaxis in acute liver failure: friend or foe? Clin Gastroenterol Hepatol 2014;12(11):1950–2.

106. Karvellas CJ, Cavazos J, Battenhouse H, et al. Effects of antimicrobial prophy-laxis and blood stream infections in patients with acute liver failure: a retrospec-tive cohort study. Clin Gastroenterol Hepatol 2014;12(11):1942–9.e1.

107. Rolando N, Philpott-Howard J, Williams R. Bacterial and fungal infection in acute liver failure. Semin Liver Dis 1996;16(4):389–402.

108. Rolando N, Harvey F, Brahm J, et al. Prospective study of bacterial infection in acute liver failure: an analysis of fifty patients. Hepatology 1990;11(1):49–53.

109. Rule JA, Hynan LS, Attar N, et al. Procalcitonin identifies cell injury, not bacterial infection, in acute liver failure. PLoS One 2015;10(9):e0138566.

110. Tujios SR, Hynan LS, Vazquez MA, et al. Risk factors and outcomes of acute kid-ney injury in patients with acute liver failure. Clin Gastroenterol Hepatol 2015; 13(2):352–9.

111. Urrunaga NH, Magder LS, Weir MR, et al. Prevalence, severity, and impact of renal dysfunction in acute liver failure on the US liver transplant waiting list. Dig Dis Sci 2016;61(1):309–16.

112. Davenport A, Will EJ, Davidson AM. Improved cardiovascular stability during continuous modes of renal replacement therapy in critically ill patients with acute hepatic and renal failure. Crit Care Med 1993;21(3):328–38.

113. Banares R, Catalina MV, Vaquero J. Molecular adsorbent recirculating system and bioartificial devices for liver failure. Clin Liver Dis 2014;18(4):945–56.

114. Saliba F, Camus C, Durand F, et al. Albumin dialysis with a noncell artificial liver support device in patients with acute liver failure: a randomized, controlled trial. Ann Intern Med 2013;159(8):522–31.

115. Ellis AJ, Hughes RD, Wendon JA, et al. Pilot-controlled trial of the extracorporeal liver assist device in acute liver failure. Hepatology 1996;24(6):1446–51.

116. Demetriou AA, Brown RS Jr, Busuttil RW, et al. Prospective, randomized, multi-center, controlled trial of a bioartificial liver in treating acute liver failure. Ann Surg 2004;239(5):660–7 [discussion: 667–70].

117. El Banayosy A, Kizner L, Schueler V, et al. First use of the molecular adsorbent recirculating system technique on patients with hypoxic liver failure after cardio-genic shock. ASAIO J 2004;50(4):332–7.

118. Larsen FS, Schmidt LE, Bernsmeier C, et al. High-volume plasma exchange in patients with acute liver failure: an open randomised controlled trial. J Hepatol 2016;64(1):69–78.

119. Reddy KR, Ellerbe C, Schilsky M, et al. Determinants of outcome among pa-tients with acute liver failure listed for liver transplantation in the United States. Liver Transpl 2016;22(4):505–15.

120. Barshes NR, Lee TC, Balkrishnan R, et al. Risk stratification of adult patients un-dergoing orthotopic liver transplantation for fulminant hepatic failure. Transplan-tation 2006;81(2):195–201.

121. Berg CL, Steffick DE, Edwards EB, et al. Liver and intestine transplantation in the United States 1998-2007. Am J Transplant 2009;9(4 Pt 2):907–31.

122. Farmer DG, Anselmo DM, Ghobrial RM, et al. Liver transplantation for fulminant hepatic failure: experience with more than 200 patients over a 17-year period. Ann Surg 2003;237(5):666–75 [discussion: 675–6].

123. Campsen J, Blei AT, Emond JC, et al. Outcomes of living donor liver transplan-tation for acute liver failure: the adult-to-adult living donor liver transplantation cohort study. Liver Transpl 2008;14(9):1273–80.

124. Uemoto S, Inomata Y, Sakurai T, et al. Living donor liver transplantation for fulmi-nant hepatic failure. Transplantation 2000;70(1):152–7.

125. Hanto DW, Fecteau AH, Alonso MH, et al. ABO-incompatible liver transplantation with no immunological graft losses using total plasma exchange, splenectomy, and quadruple immunosuppression: evidence for accommodation. Liver Transpl 2003;9(1):22–30.
126. Toso C, Al-Qahtani M, Alsaif FA, et al. ABO-incompatible liver transplantation for critically ill adult patients. Transpl Int 2007;20(8):675–81.

Follow-up of the Post-Liver Transplantation Patient

A Primer for the Practicing Gastroenterologist

Amanda Cheung, MD, Josh Levitsky, MD, MS*

KEYWORDS

- Liver transplantation • Immunosuppression • Outcomes • Prophylaxis • Screening

KEY POINTS

- Liver transplantation outcomes have improved; therefore, transplant recipients are living longer and the long-term effects of immunosuppression are becoming more evident.
- The risk of infection is greatest in the perioperative period but persists lifelong due to the use of immunosuppression.
- Long-term effects from the use of immunosuppression include metabolic syndrome, diabetes, hypertension, dyslipidemia, cardiovascular disease, renal dysfunction, osteoporosis, and malignancy.
- Liver transplant recipients require close monitoring to detect complications related to the transplant and long-term immunosuppression; regular physician visits are needed for screening and surveillance of complications.

INTRODUCTION

Liver transplantation outcomes have continued to improve, with the most recent data analysis estimating patient and graft survival rates of 92.2% at 6 months, 89.7% at 1 year, and 53% at 10 years (**Fig. 1**).[1] Until recently, the most common indication for liver transplantation has been chronic hepatitis C. With the recent advent of direct-acting antiviral therapy, the prevailing indication for liver transplantation will change in the near future, with a notable increase in nonalcoholic fatty liver disease (**Fig. 2**). Early posttransplant complications include primary graft dysfunction, acute cellular rejection, infections, hepatic artery thrombosis, portal vein thrombosis, biliary leaks, and biliary strictures. After the first year posttransplantation, modifiable risk

Disclosure: Advisor and stock holder for Transplant Genomics Incorporated; Speaker for Gilead, Salix, Novartis; Research grants from Novartis, Abbvie (J. Levitsky). A. Cheung has nothing to disclose.
Division of Gastroenterology and Hepatology, Northwestern University, 676 North Saint Clair, Suite 1400, Chicago, IL 60611, USA
* Corresponding author.
E-mail address: josh.levitsky@nm.org

Clin Liver Dis 21 (2017) 793–813
http://dx.doi.org/10.1016/j.cld.2017.06.006
1089-3261/17/© 2017 Elsevier Inc. All rights reserved.
liver.theclinics.com

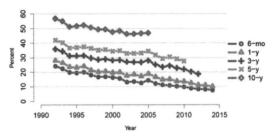

Fig. 1. Graft failure among adult deceased donor liver transplant recipients. (*Data from* Scientific registry of transplant recipients. Available at: http://srtr.transplant.hrsa.gov/annual_reports/Default.aspx. Accessed January 25, 2017.)

factors associated with higher mortality include hypertension, diabetes, renal insufficiency, and smoking. Based on data collected from the National Institute of Diabetes and Digestive and Kidney Diseases Liver Transplantation Database, the most common overall causes of death were hepatic (recurrent disease or liver failure) causes (23.9%), malignancy (18.7%), infection (15.9%), cardiovascular disease (12.2%), and renal failure (4.3%).[2] The cause of death differs in the early versus late postoperative periods, with a notable decrease in infection and increase in renal failure. In patients who survived 5 years after transplantation, the primary cause of death was attributed to hepatic causes (27.3%), malignancy (21.1%), renal failure (10.2%), cardiovascular disease (8.6%), and infection (8.6%).[2] Hepatic causes of death will likely decrease significantly in the near future since most of these deaths were related to the complications of hepatitis C recurrence; however, these cases will diminish since hepatitis C can now be successfully treated and cured in almost all recipients.

This review focuses on the complications seen after liver transplantation and the screening or surveillance needed to mitigate these complications. Malignancy, infection, cardiovascular disease, and renal failure are the most commons causes of death and should be the focus of posttransplant care.

IMMUNOSUPPRESSION

Induction immunosuppression is used by up to 25% of liver transplant centers and includes antibody therapy with antithymocyte globulin and IL-2 receptor antibodies (basiliximab and daclizumab). The main classes of maintenance immunosuppressive

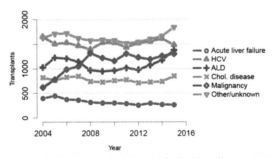

Fig. 2. Total liver transplants by diagnosis. ALD, alcoholic liver disease; HCV, hepatitis C virus. (*Data from* Scientific registry of transplant recipients. Available at: http://srtr.transplant.hrsa.gov/annual_reports/Default.aspx. Accessed January 25, 2017.)

agents are corticosteroids, calcineurin inhibitors (tacrolimus, cyclosporine), antimetabolites (mycophenolate mofetil, azathioprine), and mammalian target of rapamycin (mTOR) inhibitors (sirolimus, everolimus).

In a landmark study by the US Multicenter FK506 Liver Study Group comparing tacrolimus and cyclosporine, similar patient and graft survivals were seen with both medications, but patients receiving tacrolimus had significantly fewer episodes of acute, steroid-resistant, or refractory rejection.[3] As a result, most liver transplant centers use tacrolimus as first-line long-term immunosuppression while the other classes of immunosuppressive agents are used as adjunctive or substitutive therapy if tacrolimus cannot be tolerated due to side effects. Glucocorticoids are used in the initial perioperative period, and generally tapered off in the first year, except for patients transplanted for autoimmune liver diseases.

The selection of an immunosuppression regimen for liver transplant recipients depends on numerous factors including but not limited to age, side effect profile, indication for transplantation, presence of comorbidities, plans for conception, and history of rejection, infection, and malignancy.

Side Effects

All the available immunosuppressive agents have notable side effects (**Table 1**). Due to these significant side effects, there are ongoing research efforts to determine the feasibility of complete withdrawal of immunosuppression in carefully selected patients, although this is not yet standard of care.[4]

Drug Interactions

The calcineurin inhibitors and mTOR inhibitors are metabolized by the cytochrome P450 3A4/5 pathway and require close monitoring due to drug interactions with many commonly used medications.

Medications that increase immunosuppression levels
- Macrolide antibiotics: azithromycin, clarithromycin, erythromycin
- Fluoroquinolones: ciprofloxacin, ofloxacin
- Antifungals: clotrimazole, fluconazole, itraconazole, ketoconazole, posaconazole, voriconazole
- Antivirals: ganciclovir, valganciclovir
- Antihypertensives: carvedilol, diltiazem, nicardipine, verapamil
- Prokinetics: cisapride, metoclopramide
- Statins: atorvastatin, simvastatin
- Protease inhibitors: atazanavir, nelfinavir, saquinavir
- Proton pump inhibitors: lansoprazole, omeprazole
- Others: amiodarone, cimetidine, grapefruit juice

Medications that decrease immunosuppression levels
- Anticonvulsants: carbamazepine, fosphenytoin, oxcarbazepine, phenobarbital, phenytoin, primidone
- Antimicrobials: isoniazid, nafcillin, rifabutin, rifampicin, rifapentine
- Herbals: St. John's wort

This is not an all-inclusive list; thus, the potential for interaction with any new medication should be considered before administration.

Table 1
Side effects of immunosuppression

	Corticosteroids	Calcineurin Inhibitors		Antimetabolites	mTOR Inhibitors	
		Tacrolimus	Cyclosporine	Mycophenolate	Sirolimus	Everolimus
Diabetes	***	**	*	—	*	*
Hypertension	***	**	***	—	*	*
Dyslipidemia	**	*	**	—	***	***
Renal dysfunction	—	***	***	—	*	*
Osteoporosis	***	*	*	—	—	—
Malignancy	—	**	**	*	—	—
Teratogenic	—	—	—	***	*	*
Myelosuppression	—	*	*	**	**	**
Pulmonary fibrosis	—	—	—	—	*	*
Headaches	*	**	**	*	*	*
Gastrointestinal	*	*	*	**	*	*
Alopecia	—	*	—	*	—	—
Hirsutism	*	*	*	—	—	—

—, no known association; *, least risk; **, moderate risk; ***, greatest risk.
Abbreviation: mTOR, mammalian target of rapamycin.

LIVER-RELATED COMPLICATIONS AFTER TRANSPLANTATION
Rejection

Acute rejection typically occurs within the first 90 days but can be seen any time after liver transplantation. In an analysis from 2 large transplant databases, 15.7% of transplant recipients had at least 1 episode of acute rejection and this was independently associated with an increased risk of graft failure and death, particularly the episodes that occur more than 1 year after transplantation.[5] Patients typically present with asymptomatic elevation of liver chemistries. Although there is ongoing research to find biomarkers that may be able to predict or diagnose acute rejection, liver biopsy currently remains the gold standard for diagnosis. The key histologic features of acute cellular rejection include venous subendothelial inflammation, inflammatory bile duct injury, and portal tract mixed inflammatory infiltrates. However, differentiation between acute rejection and hepatitis from viral disease, drugs, and autoimmunity can be difficult given overlap of clinical and histologic features.[6] Treatment of acute rejection varies among transplant centers but typically includes intravenous methylprednisolone followed by a corticosteroid taper, as well as augmentation of maintenance immunosuppression.

Chronic rejection may occur in the setting of severe or recurrent acute rejection episodes, but often has an indolent course after liver transplantation.[7] Patients with viral hepatitis and autoimmune liver diseases have up to a 4 times greater risk for developing chronic rejection compared with other recipients.[8] With the advent of more effective immunosuppression, notably tacrolimus, the rate of chronic rejection has decreased to less than 5%.[9] Liver biopsy typically shows obliterative arteriopathy with bile duct injury and loss affecting more than 50% of the portal tracts. Although the early changes of arterial injury may go undetected, the damage to the bile ducts often presents with an elevation of alkaline phosphatase. Treatment of chronic rejection requires intensification of the immunosuppressive regimen. This is not always successful and may ultimately require liver retransplantation. Antibody-mediated rejection is a rare complication but can affect short-term and long-term graft survival.[10]

Vascular Complications

Hepatic artery thrombosis and stenosis may present with nonanastomotic strictures, ischemic cholangiopathy, biliary cast syndrome, or bilomas due to the dependence of the biliary tree on the hepatic artery for its blood supply. In a systematic review, the incidence of early hepatic artery thrombosis was 4.4% with a median time to detection of 7 days after transplant and a significant rate of graft loss leading to retransplantation (53.1%) and mortality (33.3%).[11] Delayed hepatic artery thrombosis occurs less frequently but with similarly poor outcomes.[12] Risk factors for hepatic artery complications include surgical technique, cytomegalovirus (CMV)-positive donor to a CMV-negative recipient, retransplantation, low recipient weight, prolonged operation time, and use of arterial conduits.[11] Portal vein and caval complications occur less frequently and are typically related to surgical technique or donor–recipient size mismatch. Treatments for vascular complications include endovascular intervention or surgical revascularization but ultimately may require retransplantation.

Biliary Complications

Bile leaks occur most commonly in the early perioperative period at the site of the cystic duct, biliary anastomosis, and cut surface in split transplantation. They can also occur immediately after T-tube removal (if used) post-operatively. Anastomotic strictures may be related to surgical technique or ischemia. Papillary stenosis may result in a biliary outflow obstruction requiring sphincterotomy. Most of these complications can be managed with endoscopic retrograde cholangiopancreatography and biliary stenting. In rare cases surgical Roux-en-Y hepaticojejunostomy revision. Non-anastomotic strictures may also be related to ischemia due to hepatic artery thrombosis. Additional risk factors include deceased cardiac donors, ABO incompatibility, Roux-en-Y reconstruction, prolonged cold ischemia time, underlying primary sclerosing cholangitis (PSC) and posttransplant CMV infection.[13] Severe cases may require retransplantation.

Recurrent Disease

Hepatitis B

Recurrence of hepatitis B infection after transplantation is nearly universal, particularly in those with high hepatitis B virus DNA levels, hepatitis B e antigen positivity, or prior resistance to antiviral therapy.[14] However, the recurrence of hepatitis B is now exceedingly rare after the implementation of prophylactic regimens using hepatitis B immunoglobulin and nucleoside or nucleotide analogues. Patients should remain on lifelong antiviral therapy to prevent recurrence.

De novo hepatitis B may occur in patients who are hepatitis B surface antigen negative and receive a liver from a hepatitis B core antibody–positive donor.[15] Similar to patients with chronic hepatitis B before transplantation, these patients should receive prophylactic antiviral medication unless they have native immunity (positive hepatitis B surface and core antibodies) and there should be little concern for hepatitis B virus transmission or related graft loss in this setting. Suggested monitoring includes hepatitis B virus DNA levels and surface antigen every 3 months for the first year and then every 6 months. Discontinuation of antiviral therapy with close monitoring may be considered if the transplant recipient has confirmed immunity with hepatitis B surface antibody.

Hepatitis C

Nearly all patients with hepatitis C viremia before transplantation will have reinfection of the new liver graft and can have an accelerated progression to cirrhosis. Risk factors associated with fibrosis progression include Caucasian race, higher hepatitis C virus RNA levels at transplantation, and use of high dose corticosteroids or lympho-depleting antibodies.[16] The most ideal time to treat hepatitis C is in the perioperative period since hepatitis C virus RNA levels are at its lowest during the anhepatic phase with viral replication starting within hours of transplantation.[17,18] Most centers will treat before or soon after transplantation to avoid detrimental histologic recurrence.

Before the advent of direct-acting antiviral therapy, treatment for hepatitis C was limited to interferon and ribavirin, which was problematic due to poor response rates, treatment toxicity, and drug interactions with immunosuppressive therapy. Approved medication regimens for hepatitis C treatment in liver transplant recipients continue to change rapidly since the introduction of direct-acting antivirals. The most updated treatment recommendations by the American Association for the Study of Liver Diseases and Infectious Diseases Society of America can be found at www. hcvguidelines.org.[19] The medications included in the currently approved treatment regimens (**Table 2**) for liver transplant recipients are ledipasvir and sofosbuvir (Harvoni), daclatasvir (Daklinza) with sofosbuvir (Sovaldi), simeprevir (Olysio) with sofosbuvir, and dasabuvir, ombitasvir, paritaprevir, ritonavir (Viekira). If protease

Table 2
Prospective HCV trials studying direct-acting antiviral therapies in liver transplant recipients

Study	Medications Used	Genotype	SVR12 Rates
ALLY-1[64]	Daclatasvir, sofosbuvir, ribavirin for 12 wk	1	95% (39/41)
		3	91% (10/11)
		6	100% (1/1)
SOLAR-1[65]	Ledipasvir, sofosbuvir, ribavirin for 12 wk	1	96% (53/55) if no cirrhosis
		4	96% (25/26) if Child-Pugh A
			85% (22/26) if Child-Pugh B
			60% (3/5) if Child-Pugh C
SOLAR-2[66]	Ledipasvir, sofosbuvir, ribavirin for 12 wk	1	93% (42/45) if no cirrhosis
			100% (30/30) if Child-Pugh A
			95% (19/20) if Child-Pugh B
			50% (1/2) if Child-Pugh C
		4	100% (7/7) if no cirrhosis
			75% (3/4) if Child-Pugh A
			100% (2/2) if Child-Pugh B
			0% (0/1) if Child-Pugh C
CORAL-1[67]	Dasabuvir, ombitasvir, paritaprevir, ritonavir, ribavirin for 24 wk	1	97% (33/34)
GALAXY[68]	Simeprevir, sofosbuvir for 12 wk	1	100% (11/11)

inhibitors are used, calcineurin inhibitor levels should be monitored closely and adjusted accordingly.

Nonalcoholic fatty liver disease
Recurrence of nonalcoholic fatty liver disease is common after transplantation. Risk factors include obesity, diabetes, hyperlipidemia, hypertension, tacrolimus-based immunosuppression, alcoholic cirrhosis as primary indication for transplantation, and steatosis in the liver graft.[20] Reported rates of recurrent steatosis (25% to 100%) and nonalcoholic steatohepatitis (10% to 37.5%) vary within the first few years after transplantation.[21] Recurrent NASH may be more aggressive in terms of fibrosis progression compared to de novo nonalcoholic fatty liver disease.[22]

The ultimate goal of therapy in nonalcoholic fatty liver disease is weight loss through diet and exercise, although the goal is often difficult to attain. Bariatric surgery in patients with NASH has been shown to improve all components of the NASH activity score to the point of complete resolution in some cases, although these patients were not transplant recipients.[23] Numerous medications with antifibrotic and antiinflammatory effects are now entering phase III trials for the treatment of NASH although liver transplant recipients are generally not eligible for the current trials. The corresponding phase II trials for each of these drugs show promising results and may soon be available for transplant recipients.

Alcoholic liver disease
Nearly all centers require a period of sobriety before liver transplantation, as well as rehabilitation and counseling. Risk factors for alcohol recidivism after transplantation include poor social support, family history of alcohol abuse, and alcohol abstinence for less than 6 months before transplant. In a metaanalysis, relapse rates were reported at 2.5 cases per 100 patients per year with heavy alcohol use and 5.6 cases per 100 patients per year with any alcohol use.[24] Although patients are at risk for recidivism, this has not been shown to increase patient or graft mortality.[25]

The 5-year patient and graft survivals in adults transplanted for alcoholic liver disease are similar to patients transplanted for other indications.[1] However, this equivalent survival does not persist beyond 5 years due to increased risk for cardiorespiratory disease, cerebrovascular events, and de novo malignancy.[25] Although all liver transplant recipients are at greater risk for de novo malignancy, the incidence rate is significantly higher in patients with alcoholic liver disease, particularly oropharyngeal and lung cancers, which may be related to substance abuse and smoking history.[26]

Patients with severe alcoholic hepatitis who have no response to medical therapy (defined by a Lille score >0.45 after 7 days of glucocorticoids) have an estimated 70% mortality rate at 6 months. Thus, waiting the typical 6 months before liver transplantation is a less feasible strategy. In a study of 26 patients with severe alcoholic hepatitis and nonresponse to therapy who were carefully selected for liver transplantation, the 6-month survival rate was 77% and 3 patients relapsed with resumption of alcohol use 2 to 3 years later but none had graft dysfunction.[27] Another smaller US study showed similar results.[28] Despite these early, positive results in very select patients (<5% of alcoholic hepatitis patients), the use of organs for this patient population remains controversial.

Autoimmune hepatitis
The reported incidence of recurrent autoimmune hepatitis is 17% to 33%.[29] Risk factors include patients with HLA DR3 or DR4 haplotype, high-grade inflammation in the native liver, or suboptimal immunosuppression.[6] Liver biopsy in conjunction with biochemical markers are needed for diagnosis, but can be difficult to differentiate from rejection. Treatment typically includes corticosteroids and increase in immunosuppression. However, more than 6% of patients will have progression of disease requiring retransplantation (hazard ratio, 4.1).[30]

Primary biliary cholangitis
Recurrence of primary biliary cholangitis (PBC) occurs in 11% to 42% of transplant recipients and is typically detected by biochemical abnormalities or protocol biopsies before symptoms (eg, pruritis, fatigue) occur.[29] Diagnosis requires histologic evaluation because the antimitochondrial antibody is not a reliable diagnostic marker after transplantation.[31] Risk factors remain unclear due to conflicting results among studies. Treatment with ursodeoxycholic acid may improve biochemical parameters, even though recurrence of PBC has not been associated with increased graft or patient survival (hazard ratio, 0.97).[32] Prophylactic use of ursodeoxycholic acid to prevent PBC recurrence seems to be a reasonable, safe strategy.[33] Patients with PBC before liver transplantation remain at risk for associated conditions, including osteoporosis and thyroid disease, even in the absence of recurrent PBC.

Primary sclerosing cholangitis
Recurrence of PSC is estimated at 10% to 37% within 5 years after liver transplantation.[29] Recurrent disease may be difficult to differentiate from chronic rejection, secondary sclerosing cholangitis, or nonanastomotic strictures related to ischemic injury. Risk factors for recurrence include HLA-DRB1*08, male gender, inflammatory bowel disease with intact colon, recurrent or steroid-resistant rejection, need for chronic steroids, and cholangiocarcinoma.[31] Risk of graft loss as a result of recurrent disease is significant (hazard ratio, 6.0).[30] Patients with PSC before transplantation and inflammatory bowel disease require ongoing screening for colorectal cancer with yearly colonoscopy, even in the absence of recurrent PSC.

Hepatocellular carcinoma

The United Network for Organ Sharing (UNOS) currently restricts transplant candidacy to patients with hepatocellular carcinoma that fulfill the Milan criteria (single tumor up to 5 cm or 3 tumors up to 3 cm each). This criteria is based on past studies that show 5-year survival rates similar to patients without hepatocellular carcinoma at time of transplant.[34] Patients within these criteria at the time of transplant had 94.5% recurrence-free survival at 5 years, whereas those outside Milan criteria had a 64.1% recurrence-free survival.[35] In the initial study describing the University of California San Francisco criteria (single tumor up to 6.5 cm or 3 tumors with a total tumor diameter up to 8 cm and largest lesion up to 4.5 cm), a more liberal classification compared with the Milan criteria, the 1- and 5-year survival rates were 90% and 75.2%, respectively.[36] Use of expanded criteria has been further studied worldwide and demonstrated some difference in the 5-year transplant survival rates for patients within or outside Milan criteria but within University of California San Francisco criteria (71% vs 85%; $P = .057$).[37]

Surveillance after liver transplantation is needed, but detailed guidance is not established. Many centers obtain cross-sectional imaging and alpha-fetoprotein levels every 6 months for the first 3 to 5 years after transplant. Patients with recurrent cirrhosis after transplant require similar screening. There is ongoing research on the use of mTOR inhibitors to decrease the risk of recurrence, although this was not proven in a large randomized trial.[38]

Infections

Liver transplant recipients are at a higher risk for both opportunistic and community-acquired infections, with the greatest risk in the perioperative period. Prophylactic use of antimicrobial agents has minimized the incidence of these infections. Nearly all patients will be placed on prophylactic agents for CMV, *Pneumocystis jirovecii*, and fungal infections immediately after transplantation. The risk of infections remains higher in patients who require higher doses of immunosuppression.

CMV viremia may clinically present with bone marrow, gastrointestinal, or liver involvement. The greatest risk for infection occurs in a CMV negative recipient and receives an organ from a CMV positive donor. Most patients receive prophylaxis in the immediate posttransplant period, typically for 3 months if the recipient is CMV positive or 6 months if the recipient is CMV negative with a CMV positive donor. After prophylactic therapy has been discontinued, patients remain at risk for CMV infection due to ongoing use of immunosuppression. A high index of suspicion is needed, particularly in patients who present with unexplained fever, cytopenias, abnormal liver chemistries, or gastrointestinal symptoms. Patients with CMV are treated with intravenous ganciclovir or oral valganciclovir until resolution of symptoms and viremia.

Risk for infections after discharge from the hospital are often related to the environmental exposures. Patients should be advised to avoid or take caution in the following settings when possible[39]:

- Persons with respiratory illnesses (viral pathogens, influenza, tuberculosis)
- Tobacco smoke (bacterial and community acquired viral illnesses)
- Marijuana smoking (fungal spores)
- Construction sites, excavation sites, dust-laden environments (spores from molds)
- Gardening, landscaping, farming, soil exposure (fungal spores)
- Animal care settings, pigeon and bird droppings, chicken coops, caves (fungal spores)

- Lake and river water, well water, untreated tap water (*Cryptosporidium, Giardia,* bacterial coliforms)
- Hot tubs (*Pseudomonas, Legionella, Mycobacteria*)
- Unpasteurized milk, soft cheese, raw or undercooked eggs (*Escherichia coli, Salmonella, Brucella, Listeria, Yersinia, Cryptosporidium*)
- Raw or undercooked meat or poultry (parasites, *Trypanosoma,* tapeworm)
- Raw or undercooked seafood (Vibrio, viruses, *Cryptosporidium*)
- Unwashed fresh produce (*Listeria, Salmonella, E coli, Campylobacter jejuni*)
- Reptiles (*Salmonella*)
- Cat litter (*Toxoplasma, Cryptosporidium, Salmonella, Campylobacter, Bartonella*)
- Birds (psittacosis, *Cryptococcus*)
- Areas with standing water (arthropod-transmitted infections)
- Outdoor activities at dawn or dusk during peak mosquito feeding (West Nile virus)

Metabolic Complications

Metabolic syndrome and its components (obesity, hypertension, diabetes, dyslipidemia) are present at a higher rate in liver transplant recipients compared with the general population due to the effects of immunosuppression and the reversal of the pre-transplant catabolic state.[40,41] The long-term effects of the metabolic syndrome are also higher in transplant patients, notably an increased risk of cardiovascular and cerebrovascular events, as well as overall morbidity and mortality.[41] Once metabolic complications are identified, patients should be counseled on necessary lifestyle modifications, including weight management, physical activity, dietary changes, and treatment of underlying comorbidities. The treatment of diabetes, dyslipidemia, and hypertension may be difficult due to the side effect profiles of the immunosuppression medications. Minimizing the doses or switching classes of immunosuppression medications may be necessary, but must be balanced with the risk of rejection.

Obesity

Obesity (body mass index $\geq$30 kg/m^2) is present in one-third of patients within the first year after transplantation. Risk factors include elevated body mass index before transplantation, presence of NASH, and presence of diabetes after transplantation.[42]

Pharmacotherapies for weight loss have limited data in liver transplant recipients. In an open-label, single arm study of 15 liver transplant recipients given orlistat, there was no significant reduction in weight and there was a possible interference with absorption demonstrated by the need for immunosuppression dose adjustments in 50%.[43] Other medications approved by the US Food and Drug Administration for weight loss (lorcaserin and phenteramine with topiramate) have not been studied in liver transplant recipients.

Bariatric surgery is an effective means of achieving weight loss and improving obesity-related comorbidities via restriction, malabsorption, and neurohormonal alteration, but there are no clear guidelines for performing bariatric surgery in liver transplant recipients. Concerns regarding a Roux-en-Y bypass surgery include the technical difficulties from prior intraabdominal surgery, potential for malabsorption of medications, and the creation of an altered anatomy that limits endoscopic access to the biliary tree. A case series of 7 patients who underwent sleeve gastrectomy at the time of liver transplantation showed that all patients had significant weight loss and no patients had diabetes, NASH, or graft loss.[44] Another case series of 9 patients who had a sleeve gastrectomy showed effective weight loss without compromising graft function.[45]

Diabetes

Patients with diabetes before liver transplantation nearly always have persistent diabetes requiring medications after transplantation. New-onset diabetes mellitus is estimated to occur in one-fourth of liver transplant recipients, with the majority occurring within 2 years of transplantation.[46] The presence of diabetes both before and after liver transplantation is independently associated with higher mortality.[47]

Immunosuppressant medications contribute to diabetes by various mechanisms, including increased insulin resistance, increased gluconeogenesis, and decreased peripheral insulin use.[41] The use of cyclosporine is associated with a lower rate of new-onset diabetes after transplantation when compared with tacrolimus, with a risk ratio of 0.6 based on a recent metaanalysis.[48] Additional risk factors for new-onset diabetes include age greater than 50 year old, African American race, body mass index greater than 25 kg/m^2, presence of hepatitis C infection, donor greater than 60 years old, and cadaveric donor.[46]

Management and goals of treatment for liver transplant recipients with diabetes parallel those of the general population. The use of corticosteroids in relatively high doses perioperatively leads to elevated blood glucose levels that often require insulin management. Patients need to be screened for long-term complications including nephropathy, neuropathy, retinopathy, and cardiovascular disease.

Hypertension

Hypertension in patients with cirrhosis is rare due to systemic vasodilatation that is present prior to transplant. However, the development of hypertension after transplantation is common due to an increase in systemic and renal vascular resistance, which is partly related to the immunosuppressive medications (calcineurin inhibitors). Thus, dihydropyridine calcium channel blockers (amlodipine, felodipine, nifedipine) are often used first in treating hypertension due to their vasodilatory effects and minimal interaction with the commonly used immunosuppressants.[49] Of note, nondihydropyridine calcium channel blockers (diltiazem, verapamil) cause increased levels of calcineurin inhibitors and should generally be avoided.

Angiotensin-converting enzyme inhibitors and angiotensin receptor blockers have indications in patients with diabetes, heart failure, or renal disease, but may be less effective early after transplantation when renin levels are relatively low.[50] Patients with established coronary artery disease or patients who are unresponsive or intolerant to calcium channel blockers should be treated with beta-blockers.[50]

Dyslipidemia

Hyperlipidemia occurs in up to 50% of patients after transplantation.[51] All classes of immunosuppressive agents have been found to increase the incidence of dyslipidemia with greater rates observed with mTOR inhibitors or glucocorticoids compared with calcineurin inhibitors.[51]

Due to the increased risk of cardiovascular disease in liver transplant recipients, treatment parameters should be congruent with those of patients with coronary heart disease or an equivalent as defined by the National Cholesterol Education Program Expert Panel on Detection, Evaluation, and Treatment of High Blood Cholesterol in Adults.[52] Patients with a low-density lipoprotein cholesterol level greater than 100 mg/dL should be advised to undertake therapeutic lifestyle changes, including physical activity, dietary modifications, and weight management. If the low-density lipoprotein cholesterol level exceeds 130 mg/dL, initiation of lipid lowering therapy should be strongly considered.

Treatment with statins must be done carefully because they inhibit the cytochrome p450 CYP3A4 pathway leading to increased levels of both the statins and calcineurin inhibitors when used concomitantly. Therefore, statins should be used at the lowest possible doses and the patient must be monitored for development of myalgias. Pravastatin and fluvastatin are the only available statins on the US market that are not metabolized by the CYP3A4 pathway.

Cardiovascular Disease

The risk of a cardiovascular event (acute coronary syndrome, cerebrovascular accident, arrhythmia, congestive heart failure, peripheral artery disease) within 10 years of liver transplantation is 13.6%, which correlates with a 64% increased risk compared with the general population.[53] Patients with the metabolic syndrome after liver transplantation are 4 times more likely to suffer a cardiovascular event.[53] Additional risk factors include dyslipidemia, diabetes, hypertension, older age, male sex, and nonalcoholic steatohepatitis.[54]

Renal Disease

In a longitudinal study of liver transplant recipients in the United States, the estimated rate of chronic renal failure (defined as a glomerular filtration rate less than or equal to 29 mL/min/1.73 m^2 of body surface area, initiation of dialysis therapy, or kidney transplantation) was 8.0% at 1 year, 13.9% at 3 years, 18.1% at 5 years, and 25.0% at 10 years.[55] Risk factors for developing chronic kidney disease include use of calcineurin inhibitors in addition to the common causes for renal failure in the general population (hypertension and diabetes). The development of chronic renal failure significantly increases the risk of death by a factor of 4.5.[55]

Modifications in standard immunosuppressive regimens may be helpful in preventing renal impairment, especially in patients with renal dysfunction before transplantation or acute kidney injury perioperatively. The calcineurin inhibitors cause increased renal vascular resistance and decreased renal perfusion. In the perioperative period, antibody induction may be used to allow for delayed introduction of calcineurin inhibitors. Preservation of renal function may be successful if a lower dose of calcineurin inhibitors is used with adjunctive therapy, including mTOR inhibitors or mycophenolate, but this benefit is not as significant after the first year posttransplantation.[56]

Similar to the general population, control of baseline risk factors is important, including glucose and blood pressure control. Patients with concomitant proteinuria, hypertension, or chronic kidney disease should be considered for treatment with angiotensin-converting enzyme inhibitors or angiotensin II receptor blockers.

Bone Health

Immunosuppressive agents decrease bone formation by osteoblasts and increase bone resorption by osteoclasts. These medications may also affect bone metabolism by reducing intestinal calcium absorption, increasing urinary calcium excretion, increasing parathyroid hormone, decreasing skeletal growth factors, and decreasing androgen and estrogen secretion.[57] The most rapid degree of bone loss occurs in the early posttransplant period, likely related to the use of high-dose glucocorticoids. Prednisone doses as low as 7.5 mg daily have been shown to cause bone loss even in the absence of other risk factors, such as age, race, gender, or menopausal state.[57] Increased bone loss leads to a significantly increased incidence of fractures, especially in patients with a low bone mineral density before transplantation.[58] Treatment with bisphosphonates should be considered in all patients with osteoporosis or recent fractures.

Malignancy

The overall incidence of malignancy in adult liver transplant recipients is nearly 12 times greater than the general population (**Table 3**) with the highest reported rates due to skin (30.5%), solid organ (38.3%), hematologic (11.3%), and recurrent (19.5%) malignancies.[59] Risk factors include the indication for transplantation

Table 3
Incidence of de novo malignancies in liver transplant patients

	All	SIR	95% CI
Hematologic			
PTLD/lymphoma	1041	52.90	56.12–49.69
Leukemia	57	5.16	6.50–3.82
Donor related	38	—	—
Solid organ			
Kaposi's sarcoma	19	53.35	32.29–83.11
Brain	65	11.59	14.41–8.77
Renal carcinoma	121	8.71	10.26–7.16
Carcinoma of vulva, perineum, or penis	32	11.23	7.65–15.83
Carcinoma of the uterus	41	1.89	1.35–2.56
Ovarian	34	3.05	2.11–4.27
Testicular	7	1.46	0.58–3.00
Esophagus	99	22.69	27.16–18.22
Stomach	65	10.90	13.55–8.25
Small intestine	27	14.44	9.52–20.97
Pancreas	128	12.08	14.17–9.99
Larynx	67	19.29	23.92–14.67
Tongue, throat	170	61.59	70.85–52.33
Thyroid	43	4.09	2.96–5.51
Bladder	109	5.80	6.89–4.71
Breast	235	4.00	4.51–3.49
Prostate	316	2.34	2.60–2.09
Colorectal	313	7.61	8.45–6.77
Liver	458	77.94	85.08–70.80
Lung	824	13.77	14.71–12.83
Others	545	—	—
Total	4854	11.55	11.88–11.23

Abbreviations: PTLD, posttransplant lymphoproliferative disorder; SIR, standardized incidence ratio.
  Data from Zhou J, Hu Z, Zhang Q, et al. Spectrum of De Novo cancers and predictors in liver transplantation: analysis of the scientific registry of transplant recipients database. PLoS One 2016;11(5):e0155179.

(hepatitis C > alcoholic liver disease > NASH > PSC > PBC) and use of immunosuppression (steroids > tacrolimus > mycophenolate mofetil > cyclosporine > sirolimus).[59]

Skin malignancies

The use of immunosuppression significantly increases the risk of skin cancers. The incidence rates of squamous cell carcinoma and malignant melanoma are 35.7 and 2.8 times higher than the general population, respectively.[60] Due to the significantly increased risk for skin cancers, patients should be educated to always use sun protection with SPF 15 or above and limit sun exposure during peak hours. Annual skin examinations are advised for all patient regardless of skin color.

Posttransplant lymphoproliferative disorder

Posttransplant lymphoproliferative disorder is the most common malignancy in liver transplant recipients with an estimated incidence of 2% to 4% and increased risk in patients greater than 50 years of age, hepatitis C or alcoholic cirrhosis, or recipients of antilymphocyte antibodies.[61] The majority of cases are associated with Epstein–Barr virus infection leading to B-cell proliferation in the setting of depressed T-cell function from immunosuppression. Lymphoma should be considered in patients who present with B symptoms (fevers, night sweats, weight loss) and unexplained lymphadenopathy or cytopenias. Treatment requires a reduction in immunosuppression. Anti-CD20 antibodies, radiation therapy, or surgery may be considered in patients who do not improve with decreased immunosuppression or patients with more aggressive disease at initial presentation.

Solid organ malignancies

The most common solid organ malignancies in descending order of frequency are lung, liver, prostate, and colorectal in men and lung, breast, colorectal, and liver in women.[59] Screening for malignancies is similar to the general population for breast cancer (annual mammography starting at 40 years old), cervical cancer (Pap smear every 3 years or every 5 years if older than 65 years old, negative human papilloma virus testing, and negative cytology), colorectal cancer (colonoscopy every 5–10 years if no history of neoplasia and more frequently depending on history of neoplasia or family history; yearly if inflammatory bowel disease), lung cancer (low-dose computed tomography scans in smokers currently or within the past 15 years who are 55–80 years old), and esophageal cancer (esophagogastroduodenoscopy in patients with Barrett esophagus or at high risk).

MONITORING AFTER LIVER TRANSPLANTATION

Patients require lifelong monitoring after undergoing a transplant (**Box 1**). Titration of immunosuppression is typically done under the guidance of the transplant hepatologist. Patients require frequent monitoring of immunosuppression trough levels. Schedules may vary among centers but typically include labs multiple times per week initially after transplantation and later spread out to labs every 3 months after stability beyond the first year. Other comorbid conditions may be managed collaboratively with the patient's primary care physician.

Polysubstance Use

Many centers require tobacco cessation before liver transplantation, but patients may start smoking again after transplant. Since there is a notably increased risk for lung cancer, head and neck cancer, and cardiovascular disease, smoking should be strongly discouraged with implementation of cessation plans. Similarly,

Box 1
Recommendations for long-term management of liver transplant recipients

Metabolic syndrome

- Advise lifestyle modifications.
  - ○ Weight management.
  - ○ Increase physical activity.
  - ○ Dietary changes: saturated fat <7% of calories, cholesterol <200 mg daily, 10-25 g soluble fiber daily.
- Treat underlying hypertension, diabetes, and dyslipidemia.
- Use aspirin for primary prevention.

Diabetes

Screening and monitoring
- Screen for new-onset diabetes every 3 months for the first year after transplantation, followed by annual screening.
- Monitor effectiveness of treatment with hemoglobin A1c every 3 months.
- Annual screening for retinopathy.
- Annual urine specimen to screen for microalbuminuria.

Treatment
- Advise lifestyle modifications.
- Treat diabetes for a goal hemoglobin A1c <7%.
- Consider changing immunosuppression from tacrolimus to cyclosporine if poor glycemic control.

Hypertension

Screening and monitoring
- Blood pressure measurements at each clinic appointment.
- Consider self-monitoring at home.

Treatment
- Advise lifestyle modifications.
- Limit salt intake.
- Goal blood pressure <130/80 mm Hg.
- Consider dihydropyridine calcium channel blockers (amlodipine, nifedipine) as first-line medications.
- Consider angiotensin-converting enzyme inhibitors, angiotensin receptor blockers, or direct renin inhibitors if patients have concomitant diabetes, heart failure, renal disease, or proteinuria.
- Consider beta-blockers in patients with coronary artery disease or heart failure.

Dyslipidemia

Screening and monitoring
- Annual fasting lipid panel.

Treatment
- Advise lifestyle modifications.
- Treat with a statin for a goal low-density lipoprotein cholesterol <100 mg/dL. If not tolerated or LDL not at goal, add ezetimibe.
- Treat triglycerides > than 500 mg/dL or triglycerides 200 to 499 mg/dL and goal LDL with omega-3 fatty acids 1000 mg 4 times a day. If not tolerated or still uncontrolled, add fibric acid derivatives.
- If dyslipidemia is persistent, consider discontinuation of mammalian target of rapamycin (mTOR) inhibitors, lowering dose of calcineurin inhibitors, or switching from cyclosporine to tacrolimus.

Kidney disease

Screening and monitoring
- Monitor renal function by calculating the glomerular filtration rate (monitoring creatinine alone is a less adequate means of monitoring for kidney disease).
- Obtain annual urine specimen to calculate a protein to creatinine ratio, particularly in patient on mTOR inhibitor therapy.

Treatment
- Reduce calcineurin inhibitors if persistent renal dysfunction (most effective within the first year after transplantation).
- Optimize glucose and blood pressure control.
- Consider kidney transplantation in patients who develop end-stage renal disease.

Bone health

Screening and monitoring
- Bone mineral density test every 2 to 3 years for patients with normal bone mineral density.
- Bone mineral density test annually for patients with low bone mineral density or on chronic corticosteroid therapy.
- Monitor 25-hydroxyvitamin D levels at least annually.
- Screen for risk factors including dietary calcium intake, 25-hydroxyvitamin D level, gonadal status (testosterone level in men, menopausal state in women), thyroid function, and medication history.

Treatment
- Calcium (1000–1200 mg/d) and vitamin D (400–1000 IU/d) supplementation for patients with osteopenia or risk factors.
- Advise weight-bearing exercise in patients with low bone mineral density.
- Bisphosphonate therapy in patients with osteoporosis, atraumatic fractures, or osteopenia with other risk factors.

Malignancy

- Annual dermatology evaluation for skin malignancies.
- Colonoscopy yearly in patients with concomitant primary sclerosing cholangitis and inflammatory bowel disease. Otherwise colonoscopy every 5–10 years.
- Abdominal imaging every 6 months in patients with hepatocellular carcinoma before transplantation for at least 5 years, particularly in higher risk patients, or patients who develop recurrent cirrhosis in the transplanted liver.
- Consider mammalian target of rapamycin inhibitor therapy in patients with hepatocellular carcinoma in explanted liver (may be more effective in low-risk patients).

Pregnancy

- Avoid pregnancy for at least 1 year after transplantation.
- Ensure stable liver function before conception and during pregnancy with close monitoring of immunosuppression levels every 4 weeks during the first and second trimesters, then weekly until delivery.
- Coordinate care with a high-risk obstetrician.

alcohol is prohibited in the perioperative period, with most centers requiring at least 6 months of sobriety before undergoing transplantation. Resuming alcohol intake may cause liver damage just as it would to a native liver and may lead to interactions with many medications. Marijuana use should also be discouraged due to the risk of fungal exposure from contamination.

Pregnancy

Although pregnancy is uncommon in end-stage liver disease, fertility is typically restored after transplantation congruent to graft function.[62] The National Transplant Pregnancy Registry guidelines recommend liver transplant recipients wait at least 1 year after transplantation to conceive and ensure stable liver function on the lowest dose of immunosuppression possible before conception. Thus, counseling on methods of contraception is important.

Other than corticosteroids, which are pregnancy category B, the remaining medications used for immunosuppression have unclear risks to the fetus and are classified as pregnancy category C (tacrolimus, cyclosporine, sirolimus) or D (mycophenolic acid, azathioprine, everolimus). In particular, mycophenolic acid should be discontinued if pregnancy is being contemplated given its known teratogenicity.

Liver transplant recipients should be managed closely with a high-risk obstetrician. Fetal mortality rates are higher in transplant recipients with an increased risk for gestational hypertension, postpartum hemorrhage, fetal prematurity, and fetal distress at the time of delivery.[63] Although rates of complications are higher than the general population, overall pregnancy outcomes are favorable.

SUMMARY

The focus in liver transplantation in the next 10 years will likely change from preventing viral disease recurrence to minimizing the toll of rejection and fatty liver disease, minimizing the complications from immunosuppression with weaning strategies, and more optimal management of long-term risks such as malignancy, cardiovascular disease, and renal failure. In addition, now that short-term results (<1 year) have improved significantly, there will be a shift toward improving long-term patient and graft survivals, and a focus on primary care preventive strategies.

REFERENCES

1. Kim WR, Lake JR, Smith JM, et al. OPTN/SRTR 2015 annual data report: liver. Am J Transplant 2017;17(Suppl 1):174–251.
2. Watt KD, Pedersen RA, Kremers WK, et al. Evolution of causes and risk factors for mortality post-liver transplant: results of the NIDDK long-term follow-up study. Am J Transplant 2010;10(6):1420–7.
3. The U.S. Multicenter FK506 Liver Study Group. A comparison of tacrolimus (FK 506) and cyclosporine for immunosuppression in liver transplantation. N Engl J Med 1994;331(17):1110–5.
4. Levitsky J. Operational tolerance: past lessons and future prospects. Liver Transpl 2011;17(3):222–32.
5. Levitsky J, Goldberg D, Smith AR, et al. Acute rejection increases risk of graft failure and death in recent liver transplant recipients. Clin Gastroenterol Hepatol 2017;15(4):584–93.e2.
6. Demetris AJ, Adeyi O, Bellamy CO, et al. Liver biopsy interpretation for causes of late liver allograft dysfunction. Hepatology 2006;44(2):489–501.
7. Demetris AJ, Murase N, Lee RG, et al. Chronic rejection. A general overview of histopathology and pathophysiology with emphasis on liver, heart and intestinal allografts. Ann Transplant 1997;2(2):27–44.
8. Jain A, Demetris AJ, Kashyap R, et al. Does tacrolimus offer virtual freedom from chronic rejection after primary liver transplantation? Risk and prognostic factors in 1,048 liver transplantations with a mean follow-up of 6 years. Liver Transpl 2001;7(7):623–30.
9. Blakolmer K, Jain A, Ruppert K, et al. Chronic liver allograft rejection in a population treated primarily with tacrolimus as baseline immunosuppression: long-term follow-up and evaluation of features for histopathological staging. Transplantation 2000;69(11):2330–6.
10. O'Leary JG, Klintmalm GB. Impact of donor-specific antibodies on results of liver transplantation. Curr Opin Organ Transplant 2013;18(3):279–84.
11. Bekker J, Ploem S, de Jong KP. Early hepatic artery thrombosis after liver transplantation: a systematic review of the incidence, outcome and risk factors. Am J Transplant 2009;9(4):746–57.

12. Bhattacharjya S, Gunson BK, Mirza DF, et al. Delayed hepatic artery thrombosis in adult orthotopic liver transplantation-a 12-year experience. Transplantation 2001;71(11):1592–6.

13. Seehofer D, Eurich D, Veltzke-Schlieker W, et al. Biliary complications after liver transplantation: old problems and new challenges. Am J Transplant 2013;13(2):253–65.

14. Adil B, Fatih O, Volkan I, et al. Hepatitis B virus and Hepatitis D virus recurrence in patients undergoing liver transplantation for hepatitis B virus and hepatitis B virus plus hepatitis D virus. Transplant Proc 2016;48(6):2119–23.

15. Bohorquez HE, Cohen AJ, Girgrah N, et al. Liver transplantation in hepatitis B core-negative recipients using livers from hepatitis B core-positive donors: a 13-year experience. Liver Transpl 2013;19(6):611–8.

16. Berenguer M, Ferrell L, Watson J, et al. HCV-related fibrosis progression following liver transplantation: increase in recent years. J Hepatol 2000;32(4):673–84.

17. Garcia-Retortillo M, Forns X, Feliu A, et al. Hepatitis C virus kinetics during and immediately after liver transplantation. Hepatology 2002;35(3):680–7.

18. Levitsky J, Verna EC, O'Leary JG, et al. Perioperative ledipasvir-sofosbuvir for HCV in liver-transplant recipients. N Engl J Med 2016;375(21):2106–8.

19. AASLD/IDSA HCV Guidance Panel. Hepatitis C guidance: AASLD-IDSA recommendations for testing, managing, and treating adults infected with hepatitis C virus. Hepatology 2015;62(3):932–54.

20. Dumortier J, Giostra E, Belbouab S, et al. Non-alcoholic fatty liver disease in liver transplant recipients: another story of "seed and soil". Am J Gastroenterol 2010;105(3):613–20.

21. Malik SM, Devera ME, Fontes P, et al. Recurrent disease following liver transplantation for nonalcoholic steatohepatitis cirrhosis. Liver Transpl 2009;15(12):1843–51.

22. Vallin M, Guillaud O, Boillot O, et al. Recurrent or de novo nonalcoholic fatty liver disease after liver transplantation: natural history based on liver biopsy analysis. Liver Transpl 2014;20(9):1064–71.

23. Lassailly G, Caiazzo R, Buob D, et al. Bariatric surgery reduces features of nonalcoholic steatohepatitis in morbidly obese patients. Gastroenterology 2015;149(2):379–88 [quiz: e315–76].

24. Dew MA, DiMartini AF, Steel J, et al. Meta-analysis of risk for relapse to substance use after transplantation of the liver or other solid organs. Liver Transpl 2008;14(2):159–72.

25. Jain A, DiMartini A, Kashyap R, et al. Long-term follow-up after liver transplantation for alcoholic liver disease under tacrolimus. Transplantation 2000;70(9):1335–42.

26. Saigal S, Norris S, Muiesan P, et al. Evidence of differential risk for posttransplantation malignancy based on pretransplantation cause in patients undergoing liver transplantation. Liver Transpl 2002;8(5):482–7.

27. Mathurin P, Moreno C, Samuel D, et al. Early liver transplantation for severe alcoholic hepatitis. N Engl J Med 2011;365(19):1790–800.

28. Im GY, Kim-Schluger L, Shenoy A, et al. Early liver transplantation for severe alcoholic hepatitis in the United States–a single-center experience. Am J Transplant 2016;16(3):841–9.

29. Edmunds C, Ekong UD. Autoimmune liver disease post-liver transplantation: a summary and proposed areas for future research. Transplantation 2016;100(3):515–24.

30. Rowe IA, Webb K, Gunson BK, et al. The impact of disease recurrence on graft survival following liver transplantation: a single centre experience. Transpl Int 2008;21(5):459–65.
31. Duclos-Vallee JC, Sebagh M. Recurrence of autoimmune disease, primary sclerosing cholangitis, primary biliary cirrhosis, and autoimmune hepatitis after liver transplantation. Liver Transpl 2009;15(Suppl 2):S25–34.
32. Charatcharoenwitthaya P, Pimentel S, Talwalkar JA, et al. Long-term survival and impact of ursodeoxycholic acid treatment for recurrent primary biliary cirrhosis after liver transplantation. Liver Transpl 2007;13(9):1236–45.
33. Bosch A, Dumortier J, Maucort-Boulch D, et al. Preventive administration of UDCA after liver transplantation for primary biliary cirrhosis is associated with a lower risk of disease recurrence. J Hepatol 2015;63(6):1449–58.
34. Mazzaferro V, Regalia E, Doci R, et al. Liver transplantation for the treatment of small hepatocellular carcinomas in patients with cirrhosis. N Engl J Med 1996; 334(11):693–9.
35. Mazzaferro V, Llovet JM, Miceli R, et al. Predicting survival after liver transplantation in patients with hepatocellular carcinoma beyond the Milan criteria: a retrospective, exploratory analysis. Lancet Oncol 2009;10(1):35–43.
36. Yao FY, Ferrell L, Bass NM, et al. Liver transplantation for hepatocellular carcinoma: expansion of the tumor size limits does not adversely impact survival. Hepatology 2001;33(6):1394–403.
37. Duffy JP, Vardanian A, Benjamin E, et al. Liver transplantation criteria for hepatocellular carcinoma should be expanded: a 22-year experience with 467 patients at UCLA. Ann Surg 2007;246(3):502–9 [discussion: 509–11].
38. Geissler EK, Schnitzbauer AA, Zulke C, et al. Sirolimus use in liver transplant recipients with hepatocellular carcinoma: a randomized, multicenter, open-label phase 3 trial. Transplantation 2016;100(1):116–25.
39. Avery RK, Michaels MG, AST Infectious Diseases Community of Practice. Strategies for safe living after solid organ transplantation. Am J Transplant 2013; 13(Suppl 4):304–10.
40. Laish I, Braun M, Mor E, et al. Metabolic syndrome in liver transplant recipients: prevalence, risk factors, and association with cardiovascular events. Liver Transpl 2011;17(1):15–22.
41. Watt KD, Charlton MR. Metabolic syndrome and liver transplantation: a review and guide to management. J Hepatol 2010;53(1):199–206.
42. Fussner LA, Heimbach JK, Fan C, et al. Cardiovascular disease after liver transplantation: when, what, and who is at risk. Liver Transpl 2015;21(7):889–96.
43. Cassiman D, Roelants M, Vandenplas G, et al. Orlistat treatment is safe in overweight and obese liver transplant recipients: a prospective, open label trial. Transpl Int 2006;19(12):1000–5.
44. Heimbach JK, Watt KD, Poterucha JJ, et al. Combined liver transplantation and gastric sleeve resection for patients with medically complicated obesity and end-stage liver disease. Am J Transplant 2013;13(2):363–8.
45. Lin MY, Tavakol MM, Sarin A, et al. Safety and feasibility of sleeve gastrectomy in morbidly obese patients following liver transplantation. Surg Endosc 2013;27(1): 81–5.
46. Kuo HT, Sampaio MS, Ye X, et al. Risk factors for new-onset diabetes mellitus in adult liver transplant recipients, an analysis of the Organ Procurement and Transplant Network/United Network for Organ Sharing database. Transplantation 2010; 89(9):1134–40.

47. Younossi ZM, Stepanova M, Saab S, et al. The impact of type 2 diabetes and obesity on the long-term outcomes of more than 85 000 liver transplant recipients in the US. Aliment Pharmacol Ther 2014;40(6):686–94.
48. Muduma G, Saunders R, Odeyemi I, et al. Systematic review and meta-analysis of tacrolimus versus ciclosporin as primary immunosuppression after liver transplant. PLoS One 2016;11(11):e0160421.
49. Textor SC. De novo hypertension after liver transplantation. Hypertension 1993; 22(2):257–67.
50. Najeed SA, Saghir S, Hein B, et al. Management of hypertension in liver transplant patients. Int J Cardiol 2011;152(1):4–6.
51. Desai S, Hong JC, Saab S. Cardiovascular risk factors following orthotopic liver transplantation: predisposing factors, incidence and management. Liver Int 2010;30(7):948–57.
52. Expert Panel on Detection, Evaluation, and Treatment of High Blood Cholesterol in Adults. Executive summary of the third report of the National Cholesterol Education Program (NCEP) Expert panel on detection, evaluation, and treatment of high blood cholesterol in adults (Adult Treatment Panel III). JAMA 2001; 285(19):2486–97.
53. Madhwal S, Atreja A, Albeldawi M, et al. Is liver transplantation a risk factor for cardiovascular disease? A meta-analysis of observational studies. Liver Transpl 2012;18(10):1140–6.
54. Albeldawi M, Aggarwal A, Madhwal S, et al. Cumulative risk of cardiovascular events after orthotopic liver transplantation. Liver Transpl 2012;18(3):370–5.
55. Ojo AO, Held PJ, Port FK, et al. Chronic renal failure after transplantation of a non-renal organ. N Engl J Med 2003;349(10):931–40.
56. Levitsky J, O'Leary JG, Asrani S, et al. Protecting the kidney in liver transplant recipients: practice-based recommendations from the American Society of Transplantation Liver and Intestine Community of Practice. Am J Transplant 2016; 16(9):2532–44.
57. Rodino MA, Shane E. Osteoporosis after organ transplantation. Am J Med 1998; 104(5):459–69.
58. Guichelaar MM, Schmoll J, Malinchoc M, et al. Fractures and avascular necrosis before and after orthotopic liver transplantation: long-term follow-up and predictive factors. Hepatology 2007;46(4):1198–207.
59. Zhou J, Hu Z, Zhang Q, et al. Spectrum of de novo cancers and predictors in liver transplantation: analysis of the scientific registry of transplant recipients database. PLoS One 2016;11(5):e0155179.
60. Garrett GL, Blanc PD, Boscardin J, et al. Incidence of and risk factors for skin cancer in organ transplant recipients in the United States. JAMA Dermatol 2017;153(3):296–303.
61. Duvoux C, Pageaux GP, Vanlemmens C, et al. Risk factors for lymphoproliferative disorders after liver transplantation in adults: an analysis of 480 patients. Transplantation 2002;74(8):1103–9.
62. Framarino Dei Malatesta M, Rossi M, Rocca B, et al. Fertility following solid organ transplantation. Transplant Proc 2007;39(6):2001–4.
63. Coffin CS, Shaheen AA, Burak KW, et al. Pregnancy outcomes among liver transplant recipients in the United States: a nationwide case-control analysis. Liver Transpl 2010;16(1):56–63.
64. Poordad F, Schiff ER, Vierling JM, et al. Daclatasvir with sofosbuvir and ribavirin for hepatitis C virus infection with advanced cirrhosis or post-liver transplantation recurrence. Hepatology 2016;63(5):1493–505.

65. Charlton M, Everson GT, Flamm SL, et al. Ledipasvir and sofosbuvir plus ribavirin for treatment of HCV infection in patients with advanced liver disease. Gastroenterology 2015;149(3):649–59.

66. Manns M, Samuel D, Gane EJ, et al. Ledipasvir and sofosbuvir plus ribavirin in patients with genotype 1 or 4 hepatitis C virus infection and advanced liver disease: a multicentre, open-label, randomised, phase 2 trial. Lancet Infect Dis 2016;16(6):685–97.

67. Kwo PY, Mantry PS, Coakley E, et al. An interferon-free antiviral regimen for HCV after liver transplantation. N Engl J Med 2014;371(25):2375–82.

68. O'Leary JG, Fontana RJ, Brown K, et al. Efficacy and safety of simeprevir and sofosbuvir with and without ribavirin in subjects with recurrent genotype 1 hepatitis C postorthotopic liver transplant: the randomized GALAXY study. Transpl Int 2017;30(2):196–208.

UNITED STATES POSTAL SERVICE®
Statement of Ownership, Management, and Circulation (All Periodicals Publications Except Requester Publications)

1. Publication Title
CLINICS IN LIVER DISEASE

2. Publication Number
016 – 754

3. Filing Date
9/18/2017

4. Issue Frequency
FEB, MAY, AUG, NOV

5. Number of Issues Published Annually
4

6. Annual Subscription Price
$281.00

7. Complete Mailing Address of Known Office of Publication (Not printer) (Street, city, county, state, and ZIP+4®)
ELSEVIER INC.
230 Park Avenue, Suite 800
New York, NY 10169

Contact Person
STEPHEN R. BUSHING
Telephone (Include area code)
215-239-3688

8. Complete Mailing Address of Headquarters or General Business Office of Publisher (Not printer)
ELSEVIER INC.
230 Park Avenue, Suite 800
New York, NY 10169

9. Full Names and Complete Mailing Addresses of Publisher, Editor, and Managing Editor (Do not leave blank)

Publisher (Name and complete mailing address)
ADRIANNE BRIGIDO, ELSEVIER INC.
1600 JOHN F KENNEDY BLVD. SUITE 1800
PHILADELPHIA, PA 19103-2899

Editor (Name and complete mailing address)
KERRY HOLLAND, ELSEVIER INC.
1600 JOHN F KENNEDY BLVD. SUITE 1800
PHILADELPHIA, PA 19103-2899

Managing Editor (Name and complete mailing address)
PATRICK MANLEY, ELSEVIER INC.
1600 JOHN F KENNEDY BLVD. SUITE 1800
PHILADELPHIA, PA 19103-2899

10. Owner (Do not leave blank. If the publication is owned by a corporation, give the name and address of the corporation immediately followed by the names and addresses of all stockholders owning or holding 1 percent or more of the total amount of stock. If not owned by a corporation, give the names and addresses of the individual owners. If owned by a partnership or other unincorporated firm, give its name and address as well as those of each individual owner. If the publication is published by a nonprofit organization, give its name and address.)

Full Name	Complete Mailing Address
WHOLLY OWNED SUBSIDIARY OF REED/ELSEVIER, US HOLDINGS	1600 JOHN F KENNEDY BLVD. SUITE 1800 PHILADELPHIA, PA 19103-2899

11. Known Bondholders, Mortgagees, and Other Security Holders Owning or Holding 1 Percent or More of Total Amount of Bonds, Mortgages, or Other Securities. If none, check box ► ☒ None

Full Name	Complete Mailing Address
N/A	

12. Tax Status (For completion by nonprofit organizations authorized to mail at nonprofit rates) (Check one)
The purpose, function, and nonprofit status of this organization and the exempt status for federal income tax purposes:
☒ Has Not Changed During Preceding 12 Months
☐ Has Changed During Preceding 12 Months (Publisher must submit explanation of change with this statement)

PS Form **3526**, July 2014 [Page 1 of 4 (see instructions page 4)] PSN: 7530-01-000-9931   PRIVACY NOTICE: See our privacy policy on www.usps.com

13. Publication Title
CLINICS IN LIVER DISEASE

14. Issue Date for Circulation Data Below
MAY 2017

15. Extent and Nature of Circulation

			Average No. Copies Each Issue During Preceding 12 Months	No. Copies of Single Issue Published Nearest to Filing Date
a. Total Number of Copies (Net press run)			299	209
b. Paid Circulation (By Mail and Outside the Mail)	(1)	Mailed Outside-County Paid Subscriptions Stated on PS Form 3541 (Include paid distribution above nominal rate, advertiser's proof copies, and exchange copies)	79	72
	(2)	Mailed In-County Paid Subscriptions Stated on PS Form 3541 (Include paid distribution above nominal rate, advertiser's proof copies, and exchange copies)	0	0
	(3)	Paid Distribution Outside the Mails Including Sales Through Dealers and Carriers, Street Vendors, Counter Sales, and Other Paid Distribution Outside USPS®	60	50
	(4)	Paid Distribution by Other Classes of Mail Through the USPS (e.g. First-Class Mail®)	0	0
c. Total Paid Distribution [Sum of 15b (1), (2), (3) and (4)]		►	139	122
d. Free or Nominal Rate Distribution (By Mail and Outside the Mail)	(1)	Free or Nominal Rate Outside-County Copies included on PS Form 3541	88	87
	(2)	Free or Nominal Rate In-County Copies Included on PS Form 3541	0	0
	(3)	Free or Nominal Rate Copies Mailed at Other Classes Through the USPS (e.g. First-Class Mail)	0	0
	(4)	Free or Nominal Rate Distribution Outside the Mail (Carriers or other means)	0	0
e. Total Free or Nominal Rate Distribution [Sum of 15d (1), (2), (3) and (4)]		►	88	87
f. Total Distribution (Sum of 15c and 15e)		►	227	209
g. Copies not Distributed (See Instructions to Publishers #4 (page #3))			72	0
h. Total (Sum of 15f and g)		►	299	209
i. Percent Paid (15c divided by 15f times 100)			61.23%	58.37%

* If you are claiming electronic copies, go to line 16 on page 3. If you are not claiming electronic copies, skip to line 17 on page 3.

16. Electronic Copy Circulation

	Average No. Copies Each Issue During Preceding 12 Months	No. Copies of Single Issue Published Nearest to Filing Date
a. Paid Electronic Copies	► 0	0
b. Total Paid Print Copies (Line 15c) + Paid Electronic Copies (Line 16a)	► 139	122
c. Total Print Distribution (Line 15f) + Paid Electronic Copies (Line 16a)	► 227	209
d. Percent Paid (Both Print & Electronic Copies) (16b divided by 16c × 100)	► 61.23%	58.37%

☒ I certify that 50% of all my distributed copies (electronic and print) are paid above a nominal price.

17. Publication of Statement of Ownership
☒ If the publication is a general publication, publication of this statement is required. Will be printed in the NOVEMBER 2017 issue of this publication. ☐ Publication not required.

18. Signature and Title of Editor, Publisher, Business Manager, or Owner

STEPHEN R. BUSHING - INVENTORY DISTRIBUTION CONTROL MANAGER

Date 9/18/2017

I certify that all information furnished on this form is true and complete. I understand that anyone who furnishes false or misleading information on this form or who omits material or information requested on the form may be subject to criminal sanctions (including fines and imprisonment) and/or civil sanctions (including civil penalties).

PS Form **3526**, July 2014 (Page 2 of 4)   PRIVACY NOTICE: See our privacy policy on www.usps.com

Moving?

Make sure your subscription moves with you!

To notify us of your new address, find your **Clinics Account Number** (located on your mailing label above your name), and contact customer service at:

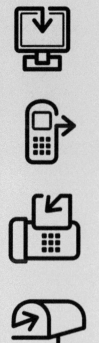

Email: journalscustomerservice-usa@elsevier.com

800-654-2452 (subscribers in the U.S. & Canada)
314-447-8871 (subscribers outside of the U.S. & Canada)

Fax number: 314-447-8029

Elsevier Health Sciences Division
Subscription Customer Service
3251 Riverport Lane
Maryland Heights, MO 63043

*To ensure uninterrupted delivery of your subscription, please notify us at least 4 weeks in advance of move.

Printed and bound by CPI Group (UK) Ltd, Croydon, CR0 4YY

03/10/2024

01040388-0017